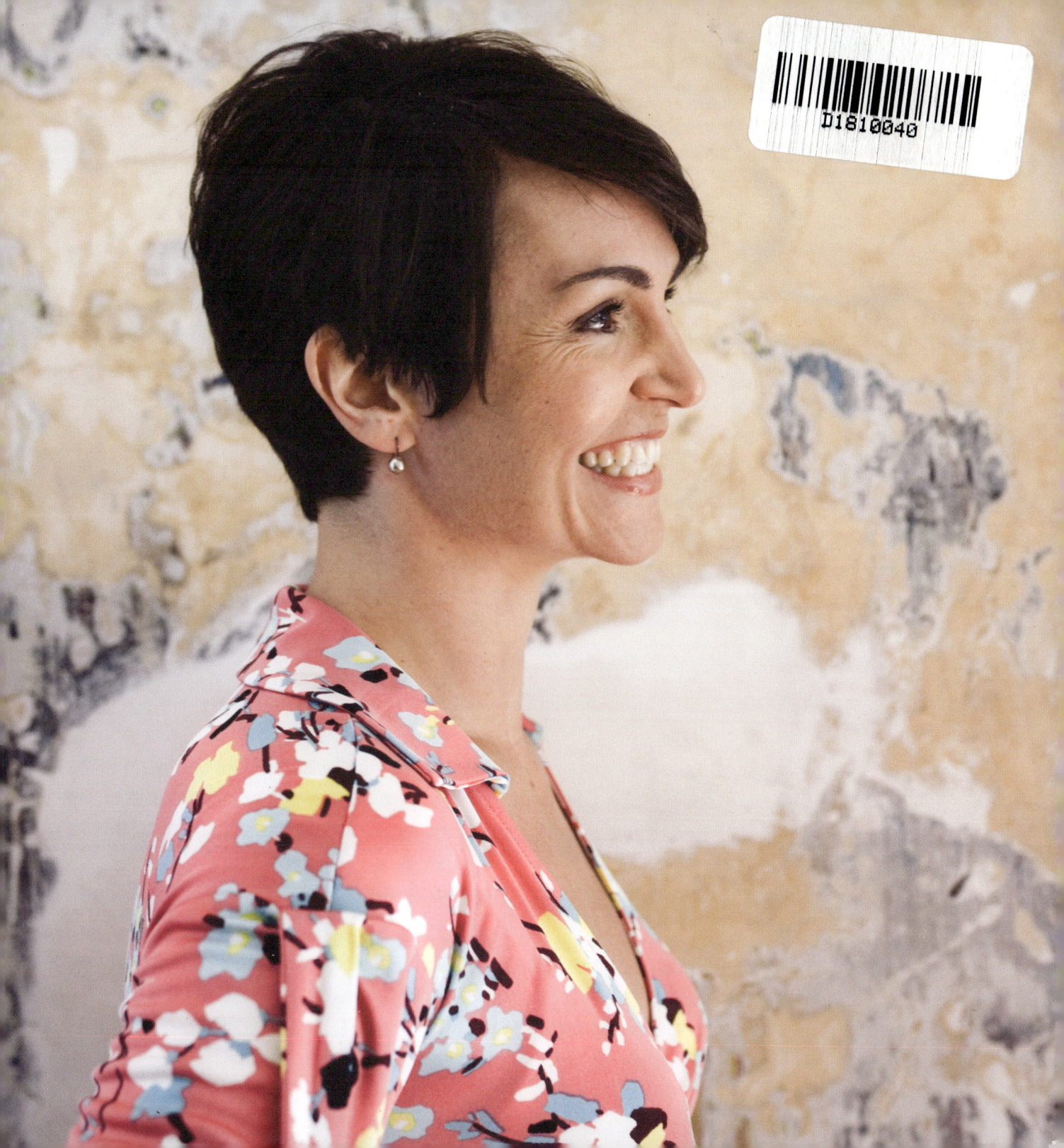

For my mum, who first taught me how to cook,
and to appreciate the importance and pleasure of
good food in life

Inner health
outer beauty

Joanna McMillan Price PhD

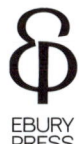

EBURY
PRESS

Contents

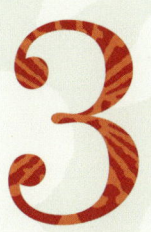
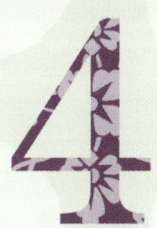

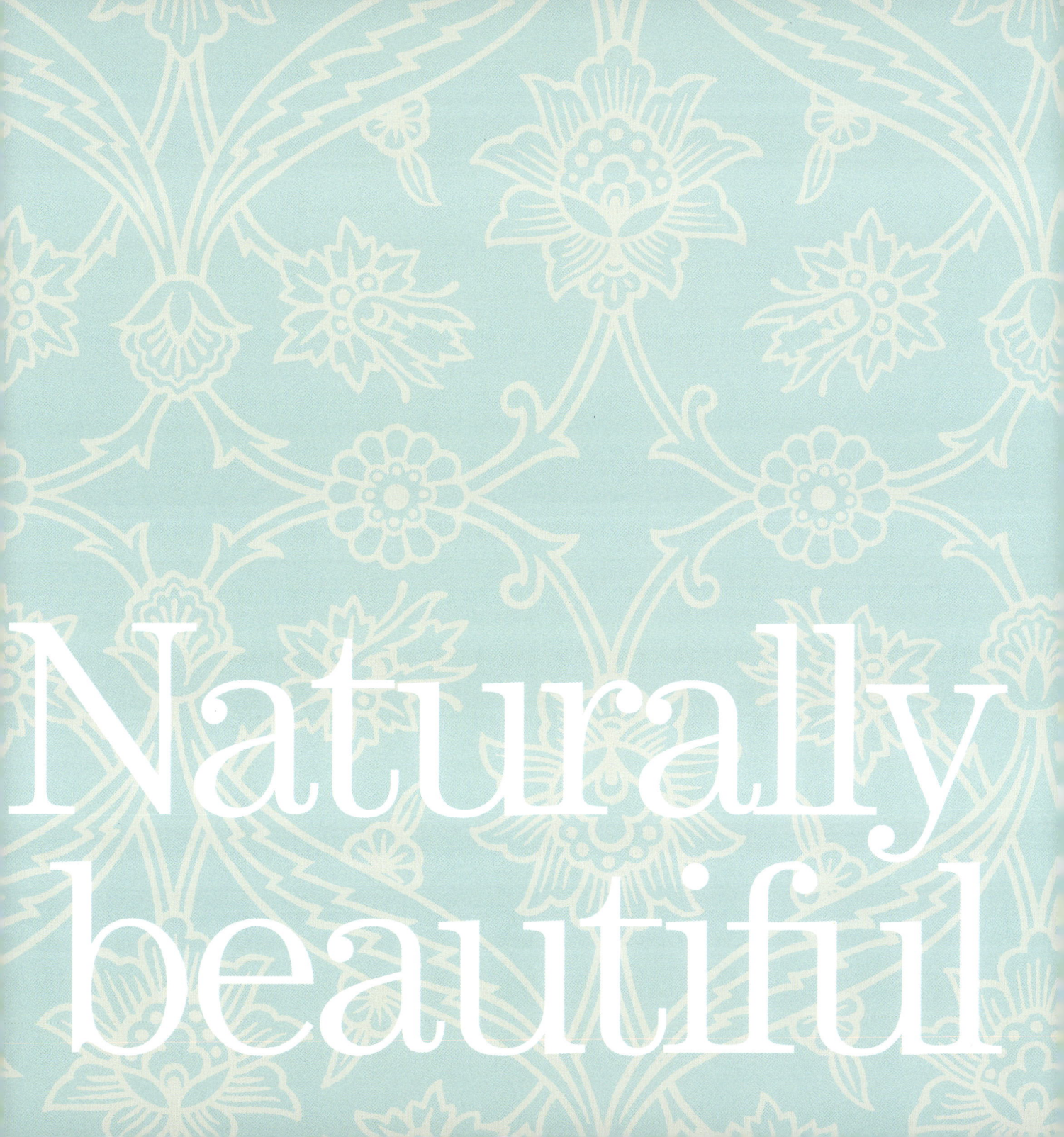

Naturally
beautiful

Many health professionals think it's the threat of chronic disease that motivates us to make changes to our diet and lifestyle. But is that true for you? Let's be honest, girls. While we all care about heart disease, cancer, diabetes and the other terrible things that can go wrong with our health, it's hard to think about those things happening to us.

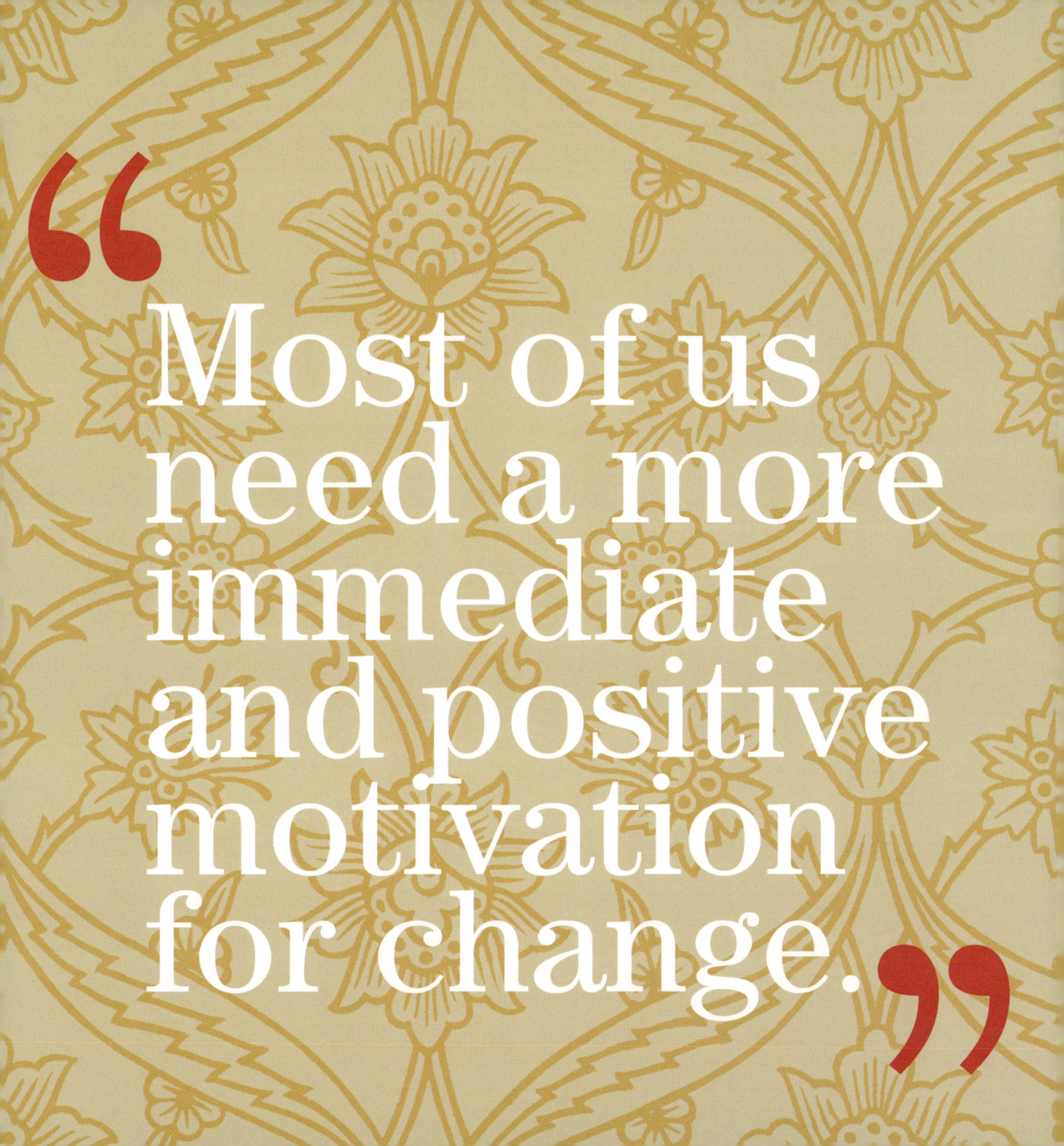

"Most of us need a more immediate and positive motivation for change."

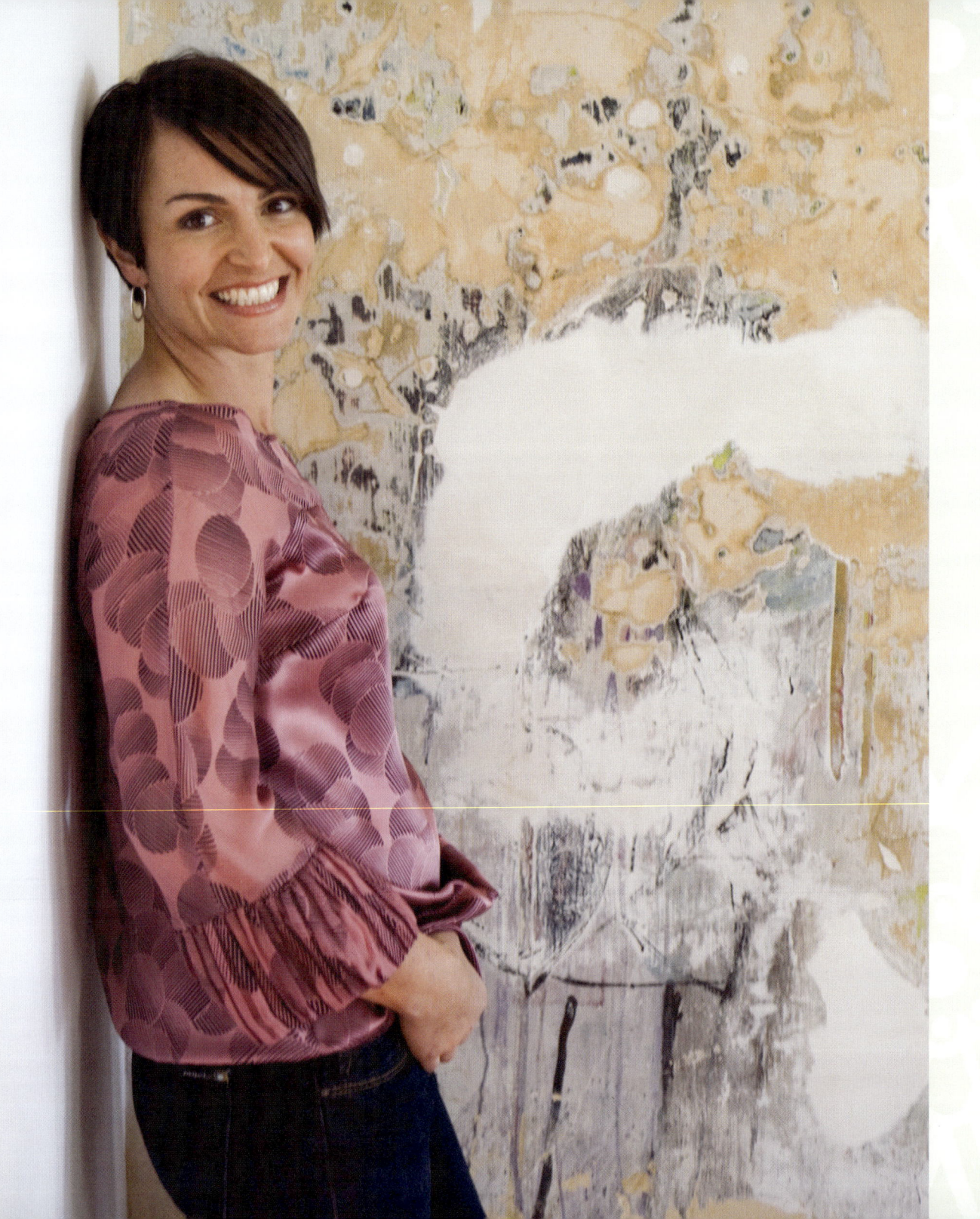

So what does motivate you?
Which of these mantras do you find more motivating?

" **I *must* eat well, exercise enough, and not smoke, or drink too much, to avoid ill health and disease.** "

Or

" **I *want* to eat well, exercise enough, and not smoke, or drink too much, to look and feel my absolute best.** "

I'm willing to bet the second mantra sounds far more appealing. Most of us want to look good, we want to look healthy, we want to have glowing skin and shiny hair, we want to have a sexy and fabulous figure, we want to slow the ageing process and, perhaps most of all, we want to feel terrific.
I'm frequently asked questions like:

'How can I eat to give me more energy while not giving up the food I love?'

'Why am I tired all the time?'

'What foods are good for my skin, hair and nails?'

'Can I lose weight without cutting out my carbs?'

'I exercise three times a week so why can't I lose weight?'

Yes, we do care about preventing disease but, day-to-day, how we look and feel is a far more powerful impetus for change.

It's all good

The good news is that the sort of diet and lifestyle changes that will help you to look and feel your best are the same changes that will help you substantially reduce your risk of major chronic disease.

Change is not easy and it's even harder to make it permanent. Here is a positive way to create the enthusiasm and motivation to help you start and stick with the plan. If I can help you to look and feel better, those immediate rewards will keep you going and motivate you to go further.

If you have picked up this book because you want to lose weight, following my principles will help you to do just that. But I want you to keep in mind all the benefits of eating the right foods. This is not a diet book with a blinkered focus on weight loss. It's a book to help women from different backgrounds and lifestyles look and feel their best. It's a book to help us all gain the benefits from eating well.

I don't mean to bag diets—there are, of course, some sound, scientifically-based ones that can be helpful. But the vast majority in the diet and health section of the bookstore are gimmicky, sold on celebrity endorsement, won't set you up for lifelong change and are often just plain boring! They don't acknowledge that food and eating are central to our social and personal wellbeing. Most importantly, they also tend to focus on weight loss, giving little thought to the nutrients you require to reap all the benefits that healthy food can bring. Weight loss at any cost? I don't think so.

As part of my research for this book I surveyed a random selection of women from several different countries and of all ages. I asked them all sorts of questions about their eating habits, how they felt about their bodies, their relationship with food and their experience of dieting. I share their responses and individual stories throughout these pages. All names have been changed to protect the respondents' privacy.

On dieting, 75 per cent of the surveyed women had been on a weight-loss diet at some point in their life. Their stories paint a clear picture of why not to follow a fad diet.

'My husband and I followed a diet that involved a lot of hard-boiled eggs. It all ended when we both got such bad piles! We did lose weight, but we then put it all back on.'
Maureen, 60s, British

'I did a New York celebrity diet book for a story I was writing. It made me feel so ill, weak, tired and completely messed up my diabetes—never again. It made me realise how unrealistic those celeb diets are. Who can actually do them in real life?' Anne, 30s, British

'I did the Israeli Army Diet with my neighbour and her mother. After two days both her mother and I gave up but conspired not to tell her daughter. On day five she was seriously sick and a doctor had to be called. All she could say was, "I don't know how you two can be feeling so great when I feel like dying!"' Suzanne, 50s, Australian

'I once went on the Israeli Army Diet with my flatmate. The second day into the green apples I felt ill and my hands throbbed... I have never felt the same about green apples!' Claire, 40s, Australian

'When my husband was alive we did do some daft diets like the Cabbage Soup Diet, which was fairly windy! My husband did a high-protein diet, which worked but was not sustainable. I have tried the Hay Diet with protein and carbohydrate days, but how can one enjoy a lamb curry without rice?'
Kirsty, 70s, British

'A friend and I did a meal replacement diet of shakes and soups—very boring, as I had to cook for the rest of the family. We had horrendous problems with constipation but we did get down to our target weights. For a while we looked and felt great but quickly put it all back on and a little more.' Lisa, 60s, British

Keeping it real

I suggest an alternative to the popular diet approach. Many of us want to and indeed should lose weight. Many more would like to tone up and lose a small amount of weight. Sixty-four per cent of the women in my survey felt they would look better if they lost a couple of kilos. For those of you happy with your figure, I'm sure avoiding weight gain is a concern, particularly as you get older. As one woman put it: 'As I've got older I've realised that I can't get away with eating anything that I want.'

So most of us are concerned about achieving and maintaining a lovely shape. But instead of it being your primary focus, I want you to put it to one side. Focus instead on the more immediate rewards of looking and feeling fabulous. If you do that and successfully eat the right foods, build a good relationship with food, adopt healthy eating behaviours and achieve the right level of activity and exercise, over time your body will *naturally* fall to (if it needs to) and stay at, the best healthy weight for you.

My equation:
Eat well + move more = look fabulous and feel great

At first glance this simple equation says nothing you didn't already know. What you have to change is your attitude to weight control. Instead of looking for a diet to provide a quick fix, consider this equation and work out what is going wrong for you. Is there an imbalance somewhere? The equation may be straightforward but it can reveal the answer to your weight woes. There is no quick fix, or at least not one that will last. What will work, however, is eating well and moving more—the weight loss will follow.

For those who are slim, don't be fooled into thinking you have nothing to worry about. Remember that weight is just one symptom of getting the diet and lifestyle balance out of whack. We can all benefit in many wonderful ways from good food and the right exercise.

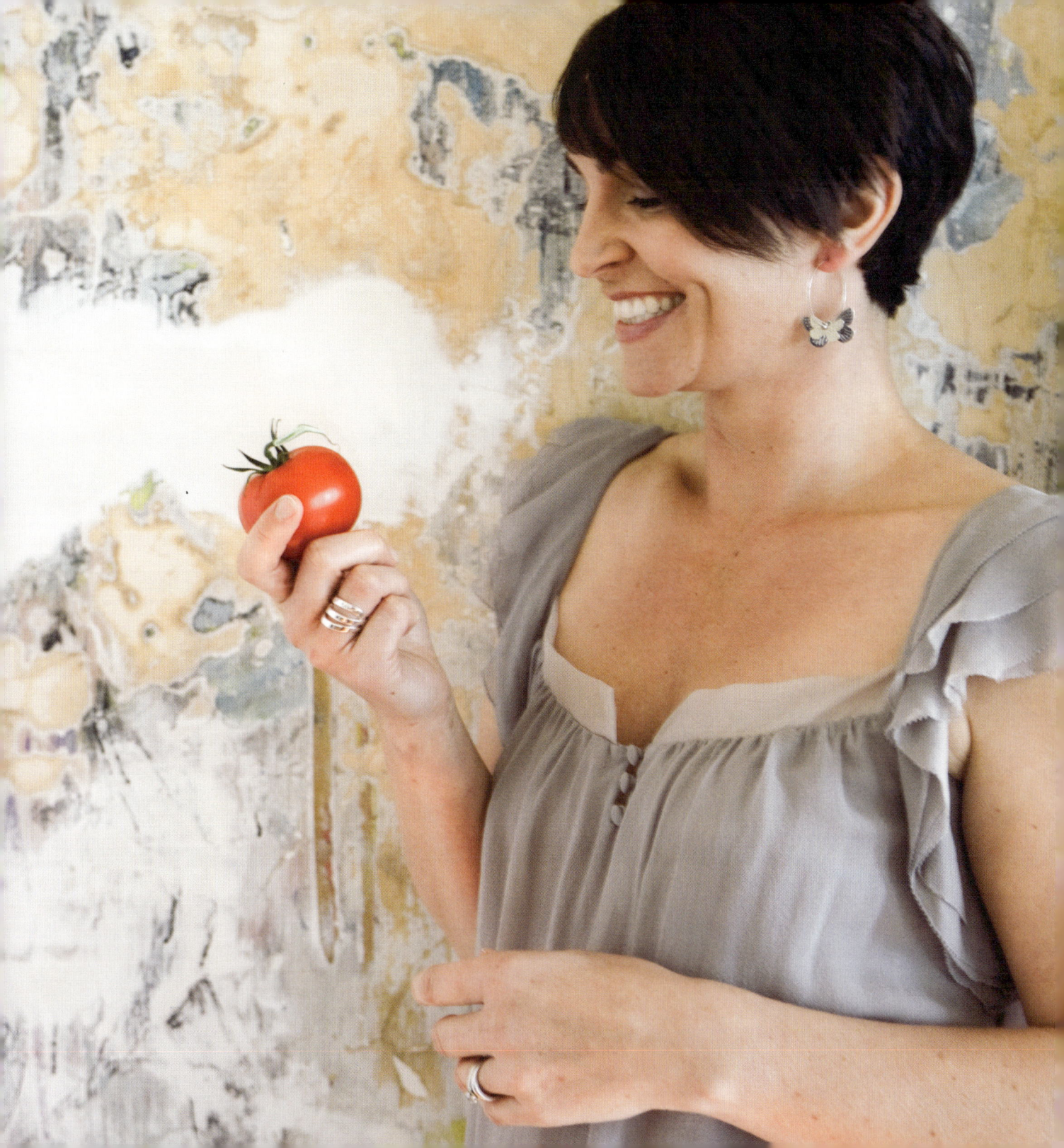

Take a fresh look at food

Until relatively recently people had few problems deciding what to eat. There wasn't much choice so they simply ate what was available locally. Today we have so much to choose from, and we are bombarded with so many different messages about what we should eat, it is no wonder that we are confused. The most common request I receive from women is an exasperated—

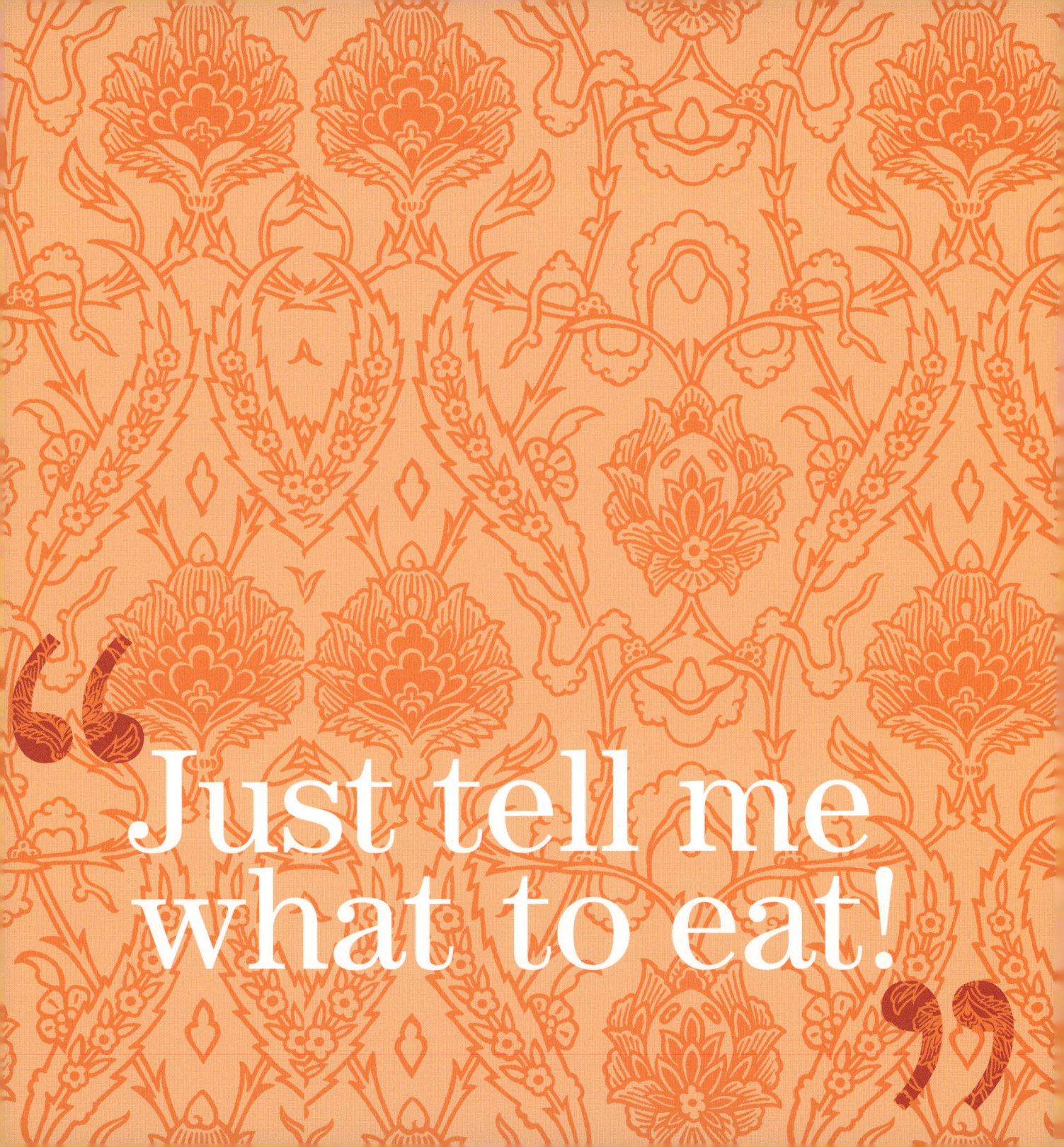

"Just tell me what to eat!"

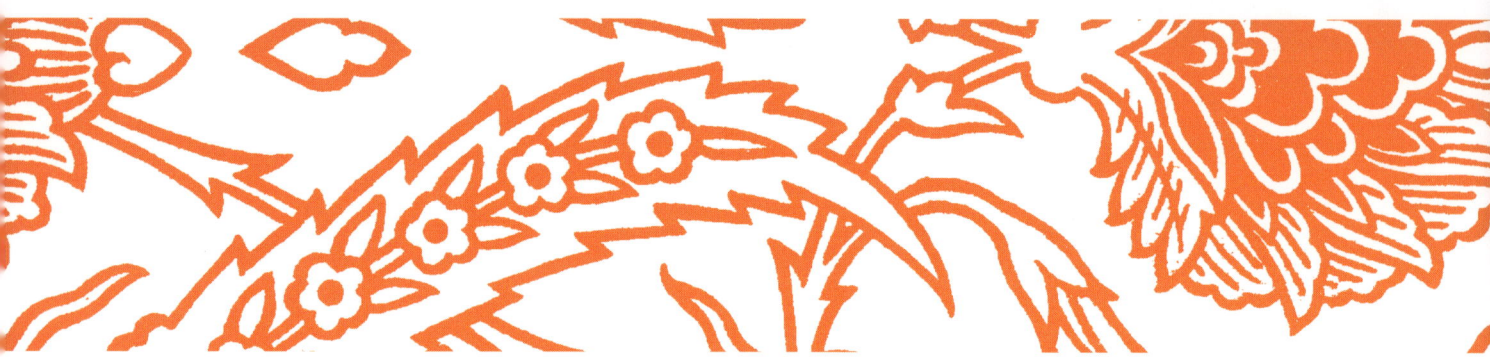

What we eat and drink affects the way we look, the way we feel and ultimately how healthy we are, now and in the future. Yes, plenty of other factors are significant, such as genetics and environment, but since we have no control over those things, let's exercise it where we can.

Eating well is not just about weight control. The right combination of food and drink can give you radiant skin, glossy, healthy hair, strong nails, clear eyes (not to mention good vision) and great teeth. In essence, if we want to look and feel our best, we have to consider what we put in our mouths.

Despite the intense scientific and public arguments over which diet is best—high protein, low fat, low GI, low carb, low kilojoule or whatever—it seems to me one message resounds above all. We do best when we go back to basics and eat real food that has been minimally processed. This is the food our bodies have evolved to eat and not the kind manufacturers have devised. I strongly encourage you to buy food as close as possible to its natural state.

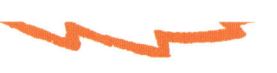
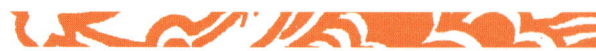

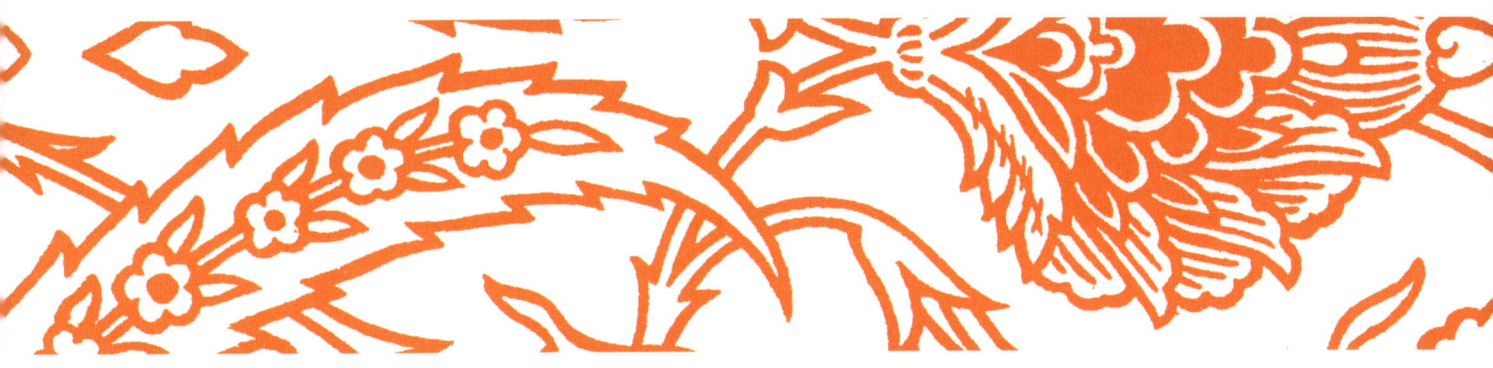

Nonetheless, we live busy lives. We don't have time most days to spend long hours buying, preparing and cooking food. Certain modern preservation, storing and food distribution techniques are convenient, safe and often necessary, and can help us achieve a healthier diet. Growing your own veggies organically in the backyard

We also now have to bear in mind more recent problems of climate change that affect agriculture; oil price hikes; and other factors that contribute to the rising cost of food. While a diet high in animal food and low in grains might be the one on which we evolved (and therefore may still physiologically be best for us), we can no longer eat that way

> **We do best when we go back to basics and eat real food that has been minimally processed.**

is commendable if you can do it, but the fact is most of us can't. What we can do instead is use selected frozen, canned, marinated and dried produce, as well as local seasonal produce, in order to eat as well as possible.

when compelling practical, ethical and environmental considerations are taken into account. The simple truth is we cannot feed the world without grains.

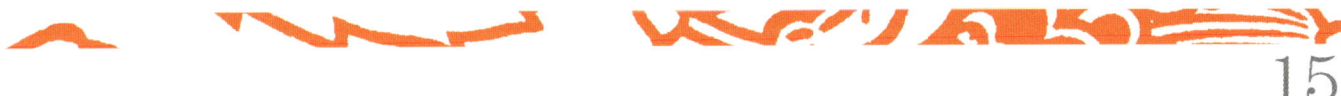

Stone Age sustenance

Let's start with a historical perspective. Far back in our ape days we probably followed an entirely vegetarian diet, as do most apes today. However, over many thousands of years we evolved into hunter–gatherers. Men, with their athletic build and growing brains, were at their iconic best—they became the hunters. Meanwhile, women fulfilled the 'gatherer' role and were responsible for everyone eating their fruit and veg. It's nice to know some things don't change! But one of the major differences between Palaeolithic girl and us is the amount of energy she expended collecting food for the family. Today, most of us drive to the supermarket and push around a trolley. The most energetic part of the whole exercise is lifting the bags into the car and lugging them into the kitchen at the other end. In comparison, our historical sisters would have spent much of the day walking, bending, stretching and lifting as they collected wild plant foods, kept an eye on the kids, and carried their 'shopping' home, most probably over considerable distances every day. And that was before any sort of food preparation began. No help in the form of pre-washed, pre-packaged salad, topped-and-tailed beans or food processors to help. It's not hard to see why our stone-age sisters weren't fat—and why so many of us are.

YOU ARE WHAT THEY ATE

Expert analysis reveals that our ancestors' diet was dominated by animal foods. These supplied crucial levels of several nutrients, including protein, omega-3 fats, iron and zinc to promote further growth of the brain and the next stage of evolution—a theory successfully played on in the Aussie adverts promoting meat, featuring the actor Sam Neill. But while our hunter–gatherer ancestors did indeed eat more protein than us, there are other major differences to consider.

Our ancestors ate

- More fibre (lots more fruit and veg): about two to three times more

- More polyunsaturated fats (from seeds and nuts) and monounsaturated fats (from olives, nuts and avocado): about one-and-a-half to two times more

- More omega-3 fats (from seafood, some plants and wild meat): about four times more

- More protein: two to three times more

- More potassium: up to three to four times more, but four to five times less sodium (more fruit and veg and less salt)

- Less saturated fat: about 60 to 70 per cent less (from butter, domesticated meats, dairy)

- No refined grains or added sugars (but they show evidence of a sweet tooth as they did eat honey) *Cardiovascular Disease* by O'Keefe, J.H. & Cordain, L. (2004)

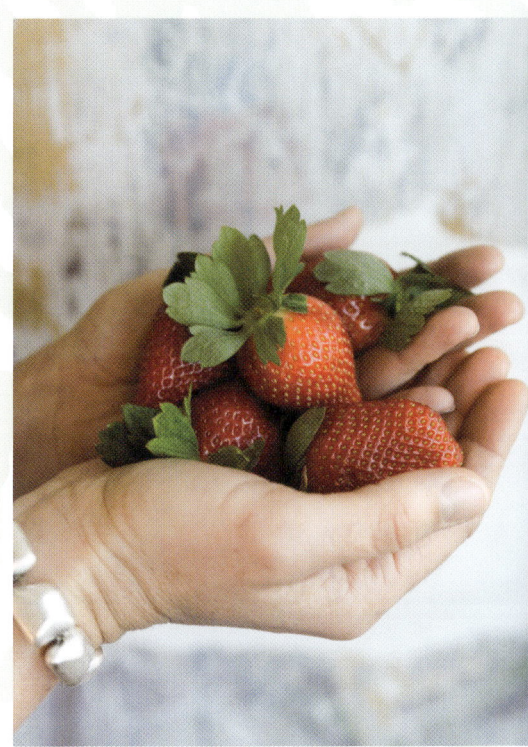

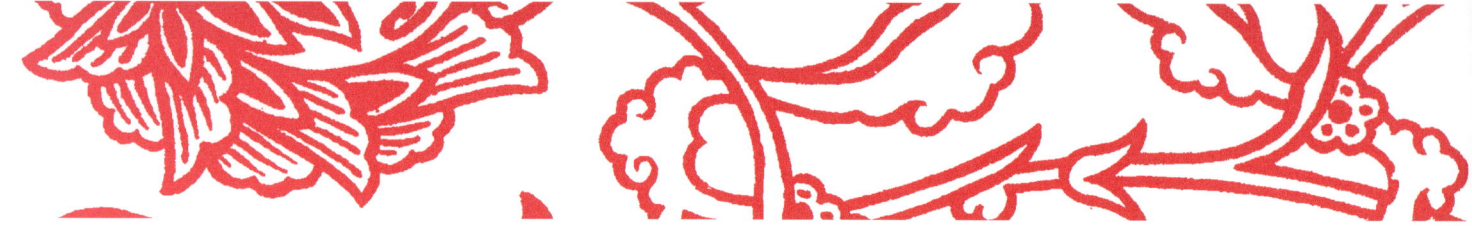

Those who tell us we should follow a high protein diet often sell their message on the grounds of it being the diet we evolved to eat. They tell us we should eat few carbs and more protein, even restricting fruits and vegetables on account of their carbohydrate content. But rarely do these modern high protein diets successfully emulate the hunter–gatherer diet. Diets that simply cut carbs and boost protein are not the way forward. The story is more complex than that, so don't eliminate foods based on their carb content alone.

Our genetic makeup has not altered since our days as hunter–gatherers. This means that although our diet has changed considerably, our bodies have not yet had sufficient time to adapt to cope with the new foods. There is a good argument to be made that we should try to eat as closely to this past diet—hence loads of books and websites espousing the 'caveman' or 'hunter–gatherer' diets. But this is virtually impossible to do.

Our ancestors ate mostly meat, lots of plant food but no grains or dairy. Shouldn't we follow genetics and do the same? Granted, their intake of animal foods was higher than ours, but the animals they ate were wild. This means they ran around a lot in their natural environment, making them lean and muscular, far more so than domesticated animals today. This affects the amount and types of fat present in the meat. The wild animals would have survived eating the foods they were designed to eat, and this too affects the fat content and even levels of certain vitamins and minerals in their meat. Let's take cattle as an example. Wild bovine relatives of the cow would have survived primarily on grass—that's what a ruminant is designed to eat. Today we want cattle to grow and fatten up as quickly as possible, and there seems to be this consensus (that I, for one, don't adhere to) that marbled meat (where the fat is all through the meat) is tastier. Feeding concentrated grain feeds to cattle helps to achieve this. Furthermore, our ancestors would also have made good use of pretty much every part of their hard-earned kill. Therefore they would have eaten many nutritious parts of the animal that you or I may not find appetising.

> " **Diets that simply cut carbs and boost protein are not the way forward.** "

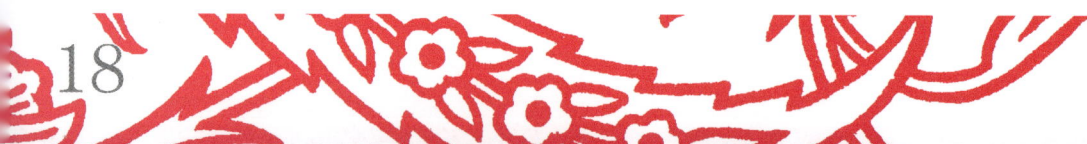

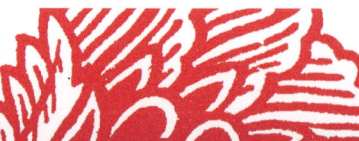

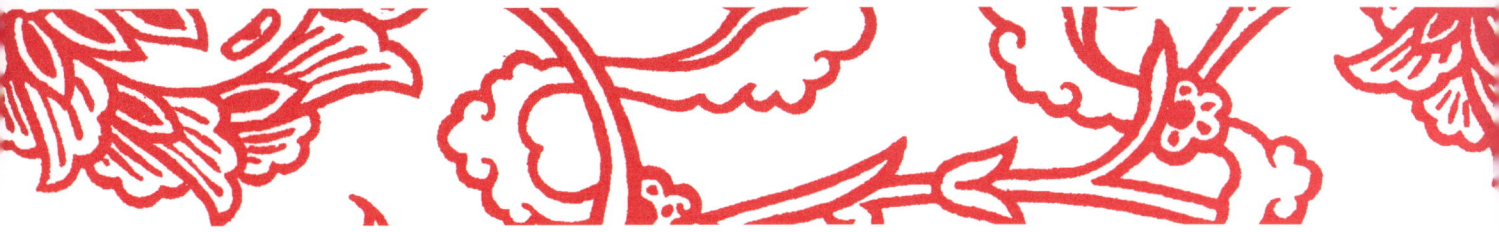

Importantly, wild prey would never have had hormone injections to promote growth (hormones are not given to chickens in this country but are used in beef cattle), been given antibiotics, nor would the meat have been treated with preservatives, with additives to make it look redder, or other modern processing techniques that have the potential to affect our health.

What about chicken? Isn't it healthier and less fatty? We are increasingly selective about which parts of an animal we eat (at least when we know what we are eating—what goes into our meat pies and sausages is a whole other story!) and like to be far removed from a connection to the living creature. For example, when was the last time you actually bought a whole chicken? For those of you who did, did you also do all the dissecting into individual parts yourself, or do you only buy one when you want to roast it whole? I'm willing to bet the latter. Most of us who eat chicken buy breasts filleted, skinned and shrink-wrapped. This means we only benefit from the nutrition in that one part of the bird. The legs and thighs have more nutrients but we have been turned off those because they have more fat. Chicken livers are used to make pâté but we rarely buy them raw to cook in other ways. None of the other chicken's organs are eaten and we miss out on boiling up the bones to make nutritious stock for use in the next meal. Our hunter–gatherer sisters could not be so selective.

What about the types of plant foods in our hunter–gatherer sisters' diet? Plants also would have been wild, and it's interesting to note that through agricultural practices we have changed the composition of some plant foods. Potatoes are a good example. The ones we buy in the supermarket almost always have a high GI, meaning that they are digested and absorbed quickly, resulting in a cascade of unwanted health effects. Many modern potatoes are also very large (think: baking potatoes). Wild species of potato are not nearly so big and tend to have a lower GI. What has happened is that by selectively breeding potato varieties to produce one that gives farmers a high yield, and produces the type of creamy, white bland flavour that food manufacturers and at least some consumers like, we have inadvertently increased their GI.

What does GI mean? The glycaemic index is a numerical ranking on carbohydrate-containing foods, based on how they affect our blood glucose levels (BGLs). Compared to a high GI food, the same amount of carbohydrate from a low GI food will result in a far smaller and gentler rise in your blood glucose. Good news for energy levels, appetite control, health of your blood vessels and control and prevention of diabetes.

GROWTH INDUSTRY

Next in our historical timeline, some 10,000 years ago, came the Agricultural Revolution. Our ancestors realised that hunting and gathering wild foods consumed an awful lot of energy. They gradually began to develop the skills to grow their own plants and keep their own animals, enabling them to have a ready supply of food. It was during this time (in some areas later than others) that we began to consume grains as we learned that seemingly inedible crops could be ground up (initially done between stones) and cooked to provide energy and nutrients. We also began to keep animals for their milk, meat and eggs. This was when dairy foods became common in many areas of the world, although not all. To this day people in Asian countries consume very few dairy products.

Over the years other common food crops have been tinkered with in a similar way to potatoes. Wheat is now one of the top three most widely cultivated crops worldwide, the others being maize (corn) and rice. It's estimated that it provides some 20 per cent of the required kilojoules of the world population. In fact, many argue that without this important crop the human race wouldn't have been able to increase its population from less than a billion about 200 years ago to an estimated 6.7 billion today. But the wheat we eat in our breads, breakfast cereals, cakes, biscuits, crackers, pasta and so on is vastly different from the ancient wheat cultivars thought to have originated in the Middle East thousands of years ago. With the invention of sophisticated agricultural machinery and processing techniques in the past hundred years, selective breeding has developed varieties of wheat that work best in the modern farming environment. This means that traits such as high yield, conformity and characteristics that allow for easy harvesting and processing of the grain have taken precedence over nutrition.

Consequently, there's been a dramatic reduction in the diversity of wheat cultivars available, as well as a change in the nutritional attributes and certainly in the taste and flavour of the grain. A number of agricultural groups, such as the Heritage Wheat Conservancy in Israel, are concerned that many of the ancient grains that nourished generations of our ancestors are being lost along with the traditional local farmers who grew them, as big corporations ship cheap, industrialised wheat worldwide.

From a nutritional point of view, many ancient grains reportedly have higher levels of protein, vitamins, minerals and phytochemicals such as antioxidants when compared to modern wheat. Some have also argued that the gluten content of modern wheat is higher than these old-fashioned varieties. This, along with the global dominance of a small number of wheat cultivars, may contribute to the increasing number of people with a dietary intolerance to wheat. This is hard to prove and the scientific literature on the subject is scant. Anecdotally, however, many people report better tolerance to the ancient grains such as spelt and kamut. These are growing in popularity as a result and are now widely available in Australia as breads, flour and pastas. You'll find them in the health food aisle of the supermarket and in whole food stores.

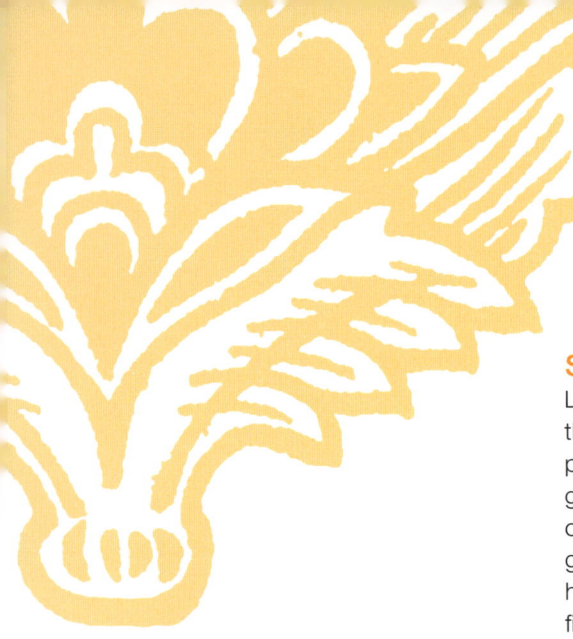

 Did you know that the French practice of consuming cheese at the end of a meal is good for teeth? The calcium and other minerals in the cheese help to remineralise the enamel, the acidity in the mouth is reduced and saliva flow is increased. All together this means less enamel erosion, fewer dental cavities and a more beautiful smile!

SO REFINED

Let's jump forward several hundred years to the Industrial Revolution for the next major change. As we devised increasingly complex machines to process food, in conjunction with developments in agriculture to produce greater crop yields, animal foods and milk, we altered appreciably the types of foods we produced. The introduction of modern milling machines allowed grains such as wheat to be broken down completely, removing the outer husk and bran layer to isolate the starchy centre. This could then be ground finely to produce an ingredient now commonplace: white flour. This process results in a massive loss of nutrients and a step-wise increase in the GI from the whole grain, to cracked grain, to wholegrain flour and finally to refined white flour.

White flour appears in so many foods it's easy to forget what a relatively recent arrival it is. We've eaten bread in some form for thousands of years, but not as we do today. Never before have we had such a pure source of energy from starch. Fluffy loaves, bagels, crumpets, pancakes, croissants, pastries, biscuits, cakes and numerous other baked foods are all newcomers to the table. I think that those who promote a low carbohydrate intake on the basis that we are not designed to eat them make the mistake of failing to recognise the difference between these modern carbs and more traditional ones. Our weight problems have risen exponentially in the past 20 to 50 years. It is not grains that are new, but the refined, processed grain foods made from them. Let's not lump all carbs together. We must eat grains to feed the world, but let's make a concerted effort to eat them in a more traditional form so we can benefit from their health-giving properties and reduce their health risks.

A way to do this is to seek out those nutritionally superior ancient grains, but regardless of which ones you choose, ancient or modern, one thing is clear: whole grains, minimally processed, are a far better choice than refined grains. The published scientific research shows that the differences between the two mean whole grains confer significant health benefits and help to prevent disease in the long term.

The whole story — whole versus refined grains

WHOLE GRAINS	REFINED GRAINS
High in fibre	Low in fibre
Good source of many vitamins and minerals	Large percentage of vitamins and minerals lost during processing, some of which are later added to compensate (but not all)
Provides phytochemicals such as antioxidants associated with good health	Phytochemicals lost with the removal of the outer layers of the grain
Digested and absorbed slowly, leading to smaller, steadier rises in blood glucose (i.e. low GI)	Digested quickly leading to large and rapid rises in blood glucose (i.e. high GI) as removal of outer husk allows rapid attack by digestive enzymes
Less insulin required	More insulin required
Filling and satiating helping to reduce total kilojoule intake	Far less filling and easy to overeat

"A generation ago, the Arab village in Sachnin, in the pastoral Galilee hills of northern Israel, produced its own indigenous, drought-hardy varieties of wheat, and 80 per cent of the men were farmers. Each morning, the fragrance of fresh bread emanated from almost every home. Today, a mere 3 per cent of the population are farmers, and more than three-quarters of Sachnin families buy mass-produced white pita bread shipped in from industrial bakeries.

Eli Rogosa, Heritage Wheat Conservancy

"The problem is what we do to food in modern

MODERN MENACES

In the past couple of decades technology has expanded even further giving us a huge influx of new foods. Fewer people create their meals from raw, whole ingredients, relying more on pre-packaged food instead. Food production has become more scientific, with complex processing plants for grains and other crops (including genetically modified ones) and chemical additives to preserve foods and increase shelf life, flavour them artificially, colour them (supposedly for greater appeal) or sweeten them without adding kilojoules. We buy food in the supermarket wrapped in plastic or packed and preserved in boxes with labels that read more like the ingredients from a chemist's lab than the kitchen.

An immense amount of energy is generated in heated scientific and public debates over the merits and demerits of high-protein or high-carbohydrate diets; whether or not we should be eating grains; whether or not meat is good or bad for us; does refined sugar contribute to chronic diseases; is milk a health food or should all dairy be cut out … the list is endless. Yet if we consider the evolutionary trajectory of our changing foods and match it to the nutritional problems we now confront, the conclusions to draw are not that complex.

When did we get fat and develop these all-too familiar major chronic diseases? It certainly wasn't 10,000 years ago when we started to eat

processing and how much we go on to eat. "

grains and dairy foods. Admittedly, several prominent scientists in the field, including Loren Cordain who writes broadly and eloquently on the subject, claim that our general health did deteriorate at this time. However, others argue that only the addition of grain foods allowed such a rapid expansion of our population. Nonetheless, our weight and chronic disease problems have escalated dramatically during the last century, particularly in the last 20 to 30 years.

Before the Industrial Revolution almost all nutritional problems were to do with 'under-nutrition'. There were famines during which people starved. Even in times of plenty there were widespread deficiencies of individual nutrients causing specific diseases such as scurvy (lack of vitamin C), beri-beri (lack of thiamine) or rickets (lack of vitamin D). Since then we have increasingly (at least in developed countries) suffered the consequences of 'over-nutrition'. We habitually eat too much, which leads to being overweight, which elevates the risks of type 2 diabetes, heart disease, metabolic syndrome, many cancers and even physical problems such as a bad back. The nature of the refined foods we eat also contributes to our risk of disease. So surely the problem is not how many carbs we're allowed, or how much protein, or whether we eat dairy foods, it's what we do to these foods in modern processing and how much of them we go on to eat.

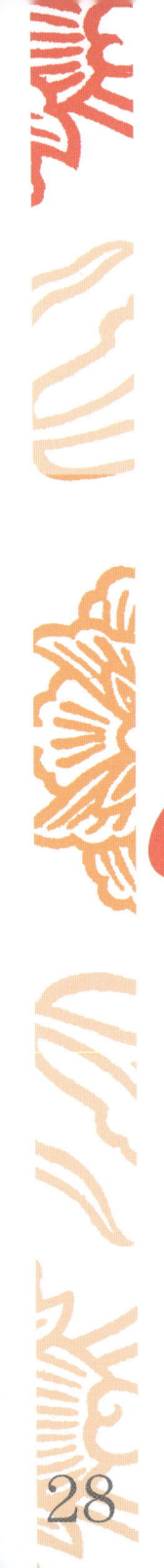

Around the world

We gain further insight into what to eat by comparing eating habits all over the world. There are many examples of dramatically different diets. The countries of northern Europe eat more potatoes and other root vegetables that grow well in cooler climates, and with a strong dairy farming tradition, butter and other dairy products feature prominently. Head further south to the Mediterranean countries and the warmer climate suits the growing of olives, grapes and other fruits and vegetables. The Mediterranean diet is rich in olive oil, a large variety of vegetables and fruits and plentiful wine. This contrasts with the very low-fat diet of the Japanese, where rice is a staple and prodigious quantities of fish and seafood are eaten, complemented by small amounts of meat. The Inuit (Eskimos), living where very few plant foods grow, eat even more fish, often parts we deem inedible, as well as whale blubber. The native diet of many African countries is almost diametrically

> "The latest predictions indicate fail to meet the life expectancy

opposed to all these other examples, based as it is on starchy plant foods such as cassava or millet with a little animal produce when it is available and affordable.

The examples are numerous and they tell us one thing: there is no single optimal diet. Nutrition scientists study the differences in disease rates between countries and consider the influence of a national diet, but this research shows many potential winners. The Mediterranean and Japanese diets are often singled out as among the healthiest, yet they differ enormously. The Inuit have low rates of heart disease yet they consume one of the highest fat diets on the planet (but 'good' fats) with limited plant food. These anomalies show us that we do not know all there is about how diet affects our health. The truth is we are highly adaptable and can thrive on any number of different ways of eating. There is, however, a common thread to these diets—they are all based on whole, natural foods. They may vary in how much animal produce is eaten, how many and what types of plant food and grains and what types of fat, but essentially they all take advantage of whatever presents itself from the water and the land.

In their fascinating book *Hungry Planet*, Peter Menzel and Faith D'Aluisio have captured what they call a 'snapshot' of the way the world eats. They photographed 30 families in 24 countries around the world with a week's worth of their usual food. The saying 'a picture tells a thousand words' was never truer. The photographs of families in more affluent countries including

... that the next generation will of their parents. "

Australia, the USA and the UK contain food items such as soft drinks, shrink-wrapped meat cuts, processed meats like bacon and sausages, processed breakfast cereals, pre-prepared supermarket meals, fast food, confectionery, packets of chips, plastic-wrapped sliced bread and packet sauces. Fresh fruits and vegetables are notably low, particularly in the US and the UK, but the two Australian families featured do not fare much better.

In stark contrast are representatives from less developed countries. For example, at least three-quarters of the foods displayed by the family in Guatemala are vegetables and fruits, they have two big bags of grains, a basket of black beans, a few raw whole chickens, a tray of eggs and very few packets. The photo from India shows a packet of two-minute noodles and a bottle of soft drink, revealing the encroaching influence of the West. Nevertheless, the bulk of foods are again in whole fresh form. At the far end of the spectrum, the family in Chad displays a fraction of the quantity of food consumed by the families in Western countries. They have a few large bowls of millet and sorghum, a few fresh fruits and vegetables that are in season, milk from their own cows, chicken and goat meat from animals they kill themselves (the goat meat is then air-dried to preserve it), and the only beverages they have are tea and water, which they collect from half a mile away.

It is clear that affluence brings many nutritional benefits. The members of the family from Chad almost certainly suffer nutritional deficiencies from a general lack of food variety, particularly from very small amounts of protein-rich foods and those animal foods that are also rich in iron and zinc. However, moving along to those countries whose populations have enough money to feed their families on a good variety of 'real' food but who don't have access to the vast array of processed foods found in supermarkets here (and even more so in the US), there is what most nutritionists would agree to be a very healthy diet. Moving to the affluent countries of the West and the health of the diet plummets. We have created more food choice, more convenience and greater availability, but at what cost? The latest predictions indicate that while up until now life expectancies have been increasing with sustained economic prosperity, the next generation will fail to meet the life expectancy of their parents.

Pulling together the historical and geographical pictures a pattern emerges. People are healthier when they consume a variety of whole, natural foods in sufficient amounts and eat few processed foods.

Lean cuisine—secrets of the Okinawans

The title for the world's longest life expectancy reportedly goes to the Japanese prefecture of Okinawa, where there is a notably high percentage of centenarians. According to the Japanese Ministry of Health, Labour and Welfare, the 2006 figures estimated there were approximately 50 centenarians per 100,000 population, compared to 10 to 20 per 100,000 population in the USA and most other developed countries. Not only do these individuals live long lives, but they also age well, with far lower rates of the usual diseases of old age, including heart disease, cancers (even stomach cancer which commonly affects the Japanese), osteoporosis and dementia.

These figures have sparked interest among researchers and the Okinawa Centenarian Study was formed in the hope of illuminating the secrets to this long-living population. The results to date highlight some interesting, although not surprising results. Firstly, the Okinawans undoubtedly possess a genetic advantage, having what the researchers have called 'human longevity genes' that place them at low risk of certain diseases. But genes don't explain the full story.

The Okinawans are very active in their daily lives (most still have jobs such as farming using traditional methods), and also take part in regular exercise, particularly in martial arts such as karate but also dancing, walking and gardening. Even in later years they remain active. They tend not to smoke and they drink alcohol in moderation. They eat lots of fruit and vegetables, including nutrient-rich seaweeds and other leafy green plants, which equals a very high antioxidant intake. They consume lots of soy—but not processed soy products that dominate our soy food choices—which contains oestrogen-like compounds that may reduce the risk of hormone-related cancers such as breast and prostate cancer. They eat lots of fish and seafood that provides them with good quantities of omega-3 fats—vital for both heart and brain health. Their diet has a low glycaemic load. Finally, and perhaps most crucially, they have a relatively low kilojoule intake. According to animal research, eating fewer kilojoules has been shown to increase life span, so it's possible that this holds true in humans also. What is certain is that obesity is a major accelerator of ageing, so the fact that the Okinawans are not fat is critical.

But the factor I think may be the most relevant of all is that they practise a cultural habit they call *hara hachi bu*, which means you only eat until you are 80 per cent full. We would do well to do the same. The Okinawans are not only lean, they are wise.

> **"There's yet another wonderful benefit to eating grains and other plant food—it's better for the environment."**

Ethical eating

In today's world we cannot make our food choices based on purist nutritional criteria. You may accept the argument that eating as closely as possible to our hunter–gatherer sisters and brothers is the best route to great health, but if we were to act that way it would be a disaster for our environment. We do not have the land available to support the farming of animals on such a scale, not to mention the methane gas production that would result. Anyone who has read Eric Schlosser's alarming book *Fast Food Nation*, or seen the subsequent feature film, will realise what major problems result from our insatiable demand for meat, particularly cheap meat. You'll never eat a commercial burger again! But while we do have to eat grains to feed the world, we don't have to eat them refined, sweetened, artificially flavoured and/or coloured or subjected to any of the other techniques used to create the junk on display everywhere we go.

This brings us to the relatively new concept of ethical eating. The organics story is part of this. Buying organic ensures your food has been produced without pesticides, artificial fertilisers, antibiotics or growth hormones in the animals and artificial additives are not added to the final product. Animal welfare promises to be better too. But ethical eating goes beyond this. It demands we think about the farmers who produce the food, the workers along the line from the farm to packaging and distribution, how the food is transported from the farm to the store and, essentially, the effect on the environment of each step on the way.

Ethical eating concerns include

- Environmental concerns
- Organic vs conventional farming
- Vegetarianism
- Sustainability, e.g. seafood
- Food miles—air and freight
- Fair trade
- Animal welfare

One aspect of the debate centres on 'food miles'. Basically this term reflects the distance food has to travel from farm to store. We're slowly getting the message that we should not buy oranges imported from the USA, even if they are cheaper, as there are enormous consequences to the environment from airfreighting them. We should instead support our own farmers and always buy Australian produce whenever possible.

Ethical eating does throw up dilemmas. Do I buy the Australian chocolate or the imported fair-trade organic chocolate? But it also helps to clear up what I call 'nutritionism gone mad'. Take goji berries as a current example. Hailed as antioxidant powerhouses with unique nutritional benefits, it seems every health food store is promoting them. However, they're flown in from the Himalayan mountains of Tibet—extra brownie points for the reader who can tell me the food miles involved there. Furthermore, there is little evidence to support those exalted nutritional claims. Given the high cost of these tiny, incredibly bland (dreadful-tasting in my opinion!) berries, we have to question who is profiting here. I'm pretty sure it isn't the Tibetans who collect the berries, allegedly by hand. A basic awareness of ethical eating immediately raises concern over such a product, sending us off to the fresh food section for some locally grown berries instead.

Nevertheless, widespread adoption of ethical eating principles requires a radical change in thinking. The average female shopper chooses her food based on price and taste. She is already more conscious of nutrition, the health effects of food, organic food … and now we have all these other considerations to take into account. Confused? Not surprising. Let's try to make things easy.

In 1961 the world's total meat supply was estimated to be 71 million tonnes. By 2007 that figure had quadrupled to 284 million tonnes and it's expected to double again by 2050. It's not just a matter of finding enough land for the farming of the animals, but also to grow the grains and soy to feed them. If we are to halt deforestation and reduce greenhouse gas emissions, is it really possible to meet this demand for meat?

Seven good food rules for life

Real food first

Eat 'real' food, in a state as close as possible to the way it is in nature. Choose minimally processed grains and grain products—brown rice over white, rolled oats over instant, muesli over sugar-coated breakfast cereal. Choose less common grains such as freekeh, quinoa or bulgur, and a wholegrain, traditionally produced bread such as sourdough. Favour whole fruit over products made with 'real fruit'. And prepare more of your own food from real ingredients rather than opting for factory-produced packaged meals.

Exit the additives

Eat food without added chemical flavourings, colourings and preservatives. The best means of ensuring this is to read the ingredient list and choose products for which you recognise all of the ingredients as individual foods. For example, consider these two tempting snacks:

Granny Annie's Hand-picked Garden Treats
Ingredients: potatoes, vegetable oils, salt

Big Hot Monster Bites
Ingredients: corn, vegetable oil, cheese powder, salt, buttermilk powder, wheat flour, whey protein concentrate, tomato powder, flavour enhancers (621, 627, 631), onion powder, whey powder, garlic powder, dextrose, sugar, emulsifier (339), food acids (270, 330), natural flavour, spices, colours (129, 150, 110)

If you read the *nutrition* label the information is almost identical—they have the same kilojoules, carbs and fat per 100 grams. But if you read the *ingredient* list, which one would you choose? It's not hard to guess that Granny Annie's Treats are old-fashioned, plain, salted potato chips. Not the healthiest food: chips are energy-dense but nutrient-poor; there is no way of telling what sort of vegetable oil was used; and the salt load is high. Nevertheless I would far rather eat these than the Monster Bites. They are a similar snack product—a cheesy corn chip—but look at the long list of ingredients, many of which are vague E numbers. Do you really know what you are eating with this 'food'? Don't get bogged down in nutrition labels, simply read ingredient lists to ensure you're not eating a cocktail of chemicals mixed with a highly refined base ingredient.

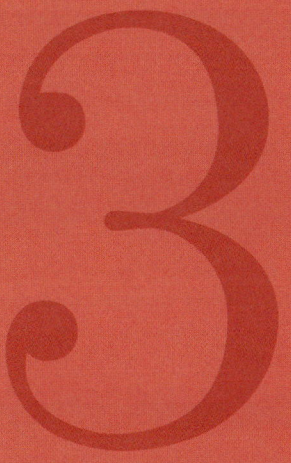

Know the locals

Eat food that is grown or produced locally as often as you can. On the face of it, it seems marvellous that we can eat many of our favourite fruits and vegetables all year round, and buy olive oil from Spain, bacon from Denmark, smoked kippers from Scotland, and mineral water from Italy. What has been lost in this mass movement of food and drink is the essence of seasonal eating. Just think of the delicious taste of your first fresh mango of summer—one of the few truly seasonal foods left in Australia. More importantly, consider the burning of fuel and subsequent environmental damage from long-haul road and air travel. We are very lucky here. We grow and produce a vast array of fruits and vegetables, we farm many grains and have thriving meat industries. We have fantastic olive oil and wines to compete with those imported from Mediterranean countries. Choosing to buy home-grown whenever possible benefits our farmers, secures greater numbers of domestic food industry jobs, maximises our chances of enjoying truly fresh produce (think of the days likely to be involved in shipping or airfreighting produce from thousands of miles away) and reduces our collective environmental footprint.

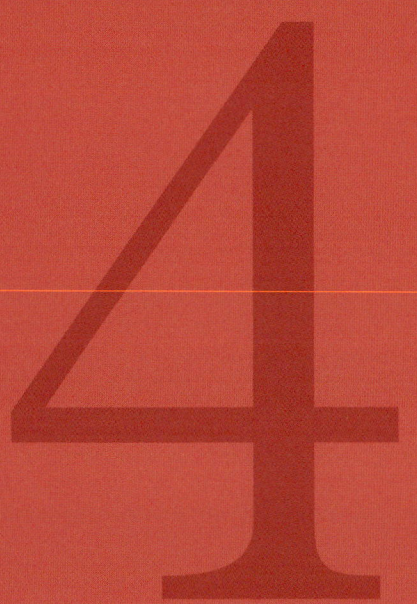

"Choosing to buy home-grown reduces our collective envionmental footprint."

4

Meat with substance

Choose meats that are as close as possible to those consumed in the past. This means lean cuts to keep saturated fat levels down while obtaining all the protein, vitamins and minerals available in animal foods. One of the healthiest and most environmentally friendly meats in Australia is kangaroo.

Another good option is grass-fed beef—if you can find it. The only grass-fed beef I have found in my area is from a premium meat butcher who sources it from Tasmania. He tells me there is a general shortage of this meat because of the drought, which has reduced the available grassland for grazing. Many people also seem to prefer marbled meat that results from fattening up cattle with grain. I appreciate that farmers must aim for high yields in order to run profitable businesses, but the current practice of feeding farm animals foods they are not designed to eat has an unfortunate effect on both the health of the animal itself and us, the end consumers. If more of us ask for grass-fed meat with any luck we can change the trend and we'll see a return to the way it is supposed to be.

5

Reconnect with nature

Give consideration to animal welfare and how meat is produced. Buy meat produced without antibiotics or hormones; free-range or organic (if you can afford it) is best. Without getting into a debate on the ethics of eating animals, most of us who do choose to eat meat like to think the animal had a happy life. We must reconnect with where our food comes from, not turn a blind eye to what happens before it appears on the supermarket shelf. Organic farming is more than food production without the use of pesticides and artificial fertilisers. It sets high standards of animal welfare and neither antibiotics nor hormones are used to promote growth. I think any one of us would agree wholeheartedly with the organic farming philosophies. The problem is that not many of us can afford to eat all organic produce, all of the time: the cost can be up to 60 per cent greater than the conventional equivalent. When choosing chicken the alternative is to buy free range—it's slightly more expensive than conventional but cheaper than organic. Free-range birds also have access to the great outdoors and have more room to move than those in a conventional chicken farm, and will not be sold as free-range if antibiotics have been used (due to illness in the bird). There are concerns that the free-range label has been abused by some large-scale egg and chicken meat producers who also produce conventional products. You can make sure of getting the best quality by buying from local small producers (often sold in your local butchers or farmer's market) as much as possible, or farms that only produce free-range.

There is an added complication with free-range eggs. According to the RSPCA many free-range farms do not provide adequate protection for birds from environmental conditions alien to them (such as hot and dry or cold and wet weather) or from predators such as foxes. In fact, the RSPCA has only accredited two free-range egg farms in the whole country. Not surprisingly, neither do they endorse the use of battery style farming of chickens for their eggs (sold as cage eggs). They do endorse free-range farms that use the 'barn laid' system. These farms keep the hens in sheds, but the birds have room to exercise, perch, nest and dust bathe—all natural activities required for their health and happiness are

It's important to change your cooking techniques when preparing lean red meat. It becomes tough and dry if you cook it at a really high heat and/ or for too long. Cook at a more moderate heat and learn to enjoy it medium–rare or rare (the meat should be soft to touch and pink in the middle).

also protected from predators and the elements. The best current means of ensuring animal welfare is to buy eggs that are endorsed by theRSPCA. Look for their logo on the box.

If you buy cage eggs because they cost less, consider that each bird shares its cage with up to four others and the cage is stacked in a large metal shed with hundreds of others. Each bird has less than an A4 sheet of paper for space and is usually de-beaked to stop it from pecking its companions in these unnaturally close-quarters. Ethically, can we support such treatment of animals in order to keep our food prices down?

Eat something fishy

As a nutritionist I have a real dilemma with fish. On the one hand I know we need to eat more of it, particularly oily fish (salmon, trout, etc.) that provide long-chain omega-3 fats essential to our health. On the other hand, our oceans are being overfished with serious consequences. Many species are already coming close to being wiped out and the wide-scale adoption of modern fishing techniques is damaging fragile marine ecosystems. I recommend you read *Australia's Sustainable Seafood Guide* produced by the Australian Marine Conservation Society to help you decide what to select. By buying our fish and seafood responsibly we can gain both the benefits of eating this fabulous food without risking the future of our precious marine system.

"The message is: quality

Go the veg

While nutritionally I support the eating of animal products, ethically, and perhaps also environmentally, I fully understand vegetarianism. But if you do choose not to eat animal products, you must take great care in planning your meals to ensure you get an adequate intake of nutrients. Include legumes, whole grains, fruits and vegetables, nuts and seeds, dairy foods and eggs (if you're not not vegan). Tofu and other soybean products are a fantastic source of protein and other nutrients and are essential in any vegan diet. The more restricted your diet, the greater risk there is of nutrient deficiencies so be adventurous. A varied plant food diet can can in fact be nutritionally better than a poorly selected carnivorous diet. However, iron and zinc are poorly absorbed from plant foods, and the crucial long-chain omega-3 fats are only present in animal food, principally fish and seafood. There are short-chain omega-3s in plant foods such as linseed, but while of benefit, these are not the same as long-chain fats. Omega-3 supplements are, of course, made from fish, so there is no easy answer here. If you are vegan you also need a supplemental source of vitamin B12. Again this nutrient is found only in animal foods, but vegetarians can buy supplements where the B12 is synthesised by bacteria.

Ultimately, the decision to become vegetarian is a personal one. But meat-eaters should also eat more plant foods and reduce their reliance on animal foods. With a few exceptions, the quality animal produce I have recommended costs more. But if we reduce our intake and bulk out our diet with more plant foods, we can still make eat in a way that is affordable and sustainable. In other words the message is: quality over quantity.

over quantity. „

What to eat

As it is crystal clear that we should avoid processed foods and eat according to ethical principles, the question remains, what do we eat to maintain excellent health and boost our natural beauty? Here are my recommendations. They form the basis of my own eating habits and be assured you will look and feel fantastic if you make them the basis of yours.

Vegetables and fruits Eat these principally because they contain loads of nutrients but few calories. So you get the vitamins, minerals, antioxidants and other phytochemicals (read: plant chemicals) your body needs to look and feel its best without the calories to add fat to your waist, hips or thighs. The greater the variety and colour the better. Eat cooked and raw fruit and veggies for maximal benefit. While good quality fresh produce is hard to beat on taste, there are many economical and convenient alternatives such as frozen produce (often more nutritious, although the taste and the texture can be affected), marinated veggies in healthy oils, fruits packaged in pure fruit juice, dried fruits (choose organic or those clearly labelled 'chemical-free' to avoid sulphite preservatives) and canned produce with no undesirable additives (canned tomatoes are a staple in my pantry but only those with 'tomatoes' in the ingredients list—harder than you might think!).

Whole grains These are among the best plant sources of energy (primarily from carbohydrates) and fibre, and they also contain good levels of protein and many vitamins and minerals. The less processed they are the better, so choose wholegrain varieties where possible. When it comes to breads, go for those that use traditional techniques such as sourdough or stone ground breads. They may be more expensive but that is because they take longer to make and use quality ingredients. The majority of modern supermarket breads use bleached flours and have added preservatives, mould inhibitors and flour improvers. Include a variety of different grains and get out of the 'bread, potatoes, pasta and rice' rut. There are a many nutritious grains to try including barley, rye, oats, quinoa (pronounced keen-wah), freekeh, buckwheat, spelt and kamut. Each has different benefits and often higher levels of specific nutrients than mass-produced grain foods.

Fish and seafood Not only do fish and seafood provide those essential omega-3 fats, they also contain many minerals that are often low in women's diets, including iron, zinc and iodine. Furthermore, they are low in the saturated fats we should avoid—and they are quick to cook and taste divine! Be careful to select in accordance with *The Sustainable Seafood Guide*.

Lean meat Remember, quality over quantity, choose the leanest cuts you can afford and, where possible, buy grass-fed or free range meat. Although not everyone likes the idea, kangaroo is undoubtedly the healthiest, cheapest and greenest meat we have. It is organic and free range; it is lean and rich in minerals (including iron and zinc); and it is a good source of omega-3 fats. Moreover, kangaroos are not ruminants and, unlike cattle and sheep, produce no methane gas. If we all swapped some of our other meats for kangaroo we could cut greenhouse gas emissions. They are also soft-footed and cause less damage to the land, are better adapted to our frequent droughts and require less food than cattle or sheep. It makes sense that a native animal would be best suited to Australia's climate and kangaroo might just be the best meat for us to eat.

Eggs What could be more natural and unprocessed? Eggs are also one of the most complete foods around, meaning they contain many of the essential nutrients we need. Yes, they contain small amounts of cholesterol, but unless you plan to eat a carton a day, it's not a problem. There is little evidence to support the notion that we should restrict egg intake at all and I would recommend one for breakfast over factory-made cereal any morning.

Nuts and seeds These are packed with energy so a few go a long way. But despite their high calorie load it has not been proven that they contribute to weight problems—on the contrary, evidence is emerging that they may do the opposite. They are rich in all the right types of fat, provide numerous essential vitamins, minerals and antioxidants and are rich in fibre. Be careful to buy them raw and not roasted in oil and drowned in salt. Nut butters without added oil, salt and sugar (particularly watch this with peanut butters) are delicious on toast instead of regular butter and are an easy way to replace unhealthy fat with the type that will do you good. There are several delectable nut spreads available, including hazelnut, almond and cashew.

Legumes Lentils, dried beans and chickpeas are good, cheap plant sources of protein, and can help to reduce our reliance on animal produce. Furthermore, they are low GI, providing slow-release carbs to fill us up while avoiding blood sugar swings. You can buy them canned for convenience (preferably not in plastic-lined cans which can leach chemicals) or dried for cooking yourself. Soybeans and the traditional foods made from them, including tofu and tempeh, are particularly high in protein. Uniquely for plant foods, they provide all of the essential amino acids (those that our bodies cannot make and which we have to eat). So if you're a vegetarian or vegan, these nutritional powerhouses are invaluable for a balanced diet.

Dairy products Not for everyone, of course, as many people have allergies or intolerances to dairy foods, but for those of us who don't, good-quality dairy is an important addition to our diets. These foods are high in protein and unbeatable for calcium. Admittedly, they are high in saturated fat, so choose low-fat varieties for everyday, particularly for milk if you consume a cup or more a day. Be careful with cheese—it's a major source of saturated fat and is easy to over-consume, particularly if you are vegetarian. Go for a traditionally produced cheese for a rich flavour minus undesirable additives. Low-fat versions are often so bland that you eat much more of them and are still not satisfied. They also contain additives to replace the function and flavour of the fat. A little of the real thing works for the French and their habit of eating a little cheese at the end of a meal is also good for teeth, helping to neutralise acids and re-mineralise the tooth surface.

Good-quality cold-pressed oils and fats These include traditional, tried-and-tested oils such as olive oil; camellia tea oil (a staple of China and other Asian countries for thousands of years, and available in the health food aisle of major supermarkets and wholefood shops); nut oils (great for salad dressings or drizzling over steamed vegetables); and, perhaps surprisingly,

✳ **Beware processed foods made from soy! These are not the same as whole soy products and the foods made from them. 'Isolated soy protein' is a cheap, processed means of adding protein to food products and has made its way into all sorts of supermarket foods. Eat soy as the Asians do and not how Western food factories have abused it.**

coconut 'oil'. Coconut fat is notoriously highly saturated and is usually found on the 'bad fat' list of the health campaign literature. This oversimplifies the fat and cholesterol issue. Not all saturated fats raise cholesterol and those found in abundance in coconut oil fall into this category. They are medium-chain triglycerides that seem to be readily used as fuel by the body and do not raise cholesterol levels. Coconut oil has many advantages for cooking because it is far more stable than highly unsaturated fats. It is suitable for high-heat cooking such as in stir-fries and in browning meat for a curry. Steer clear of highly refined (which just means filtered using chemicals), cheap oils, even if they say they are the new healthy oil.

Good-quality packaged or pre-prepared food There is nothing wrong with a few packaged foods alongside the good stuff to make life easier. These include condiments such as chutney, jam, various sauces and mayonnaise, curry pastes, soup, filled pasta and ready meals. However, no matter what food it is, if it comes in a packet, read the ingredients list. If it's relatively short with a list of recognisable foods (ingredients you could buy and use at home) then it is probably an OK, or even a good, choice. If it includes items that sound as if they belong in the laboratory, or a number of colours, flavours and preservatives that may or may not have their E number displayed, don't buy it. Aim to buy food that looks as close to homemade as possible. It really is that simple. Often the best examples come from smaller, local companies.

Good reasons to eat the right foods

- To make your skin bloom and reduce the symptoms of eczema, psoriasis and acne

- To improve the texture and look of your hair

- To strengthen your nails

- To boost your energy levels

- To elevate your mood

- To protect your teeth from cavities, enamel erosion and staining

- To bolster your immune system

- To promote a healthy gut and reduce common unpleasant symptoms such as bloating, constipation and heartburn

- To shed body fat and improve your figure

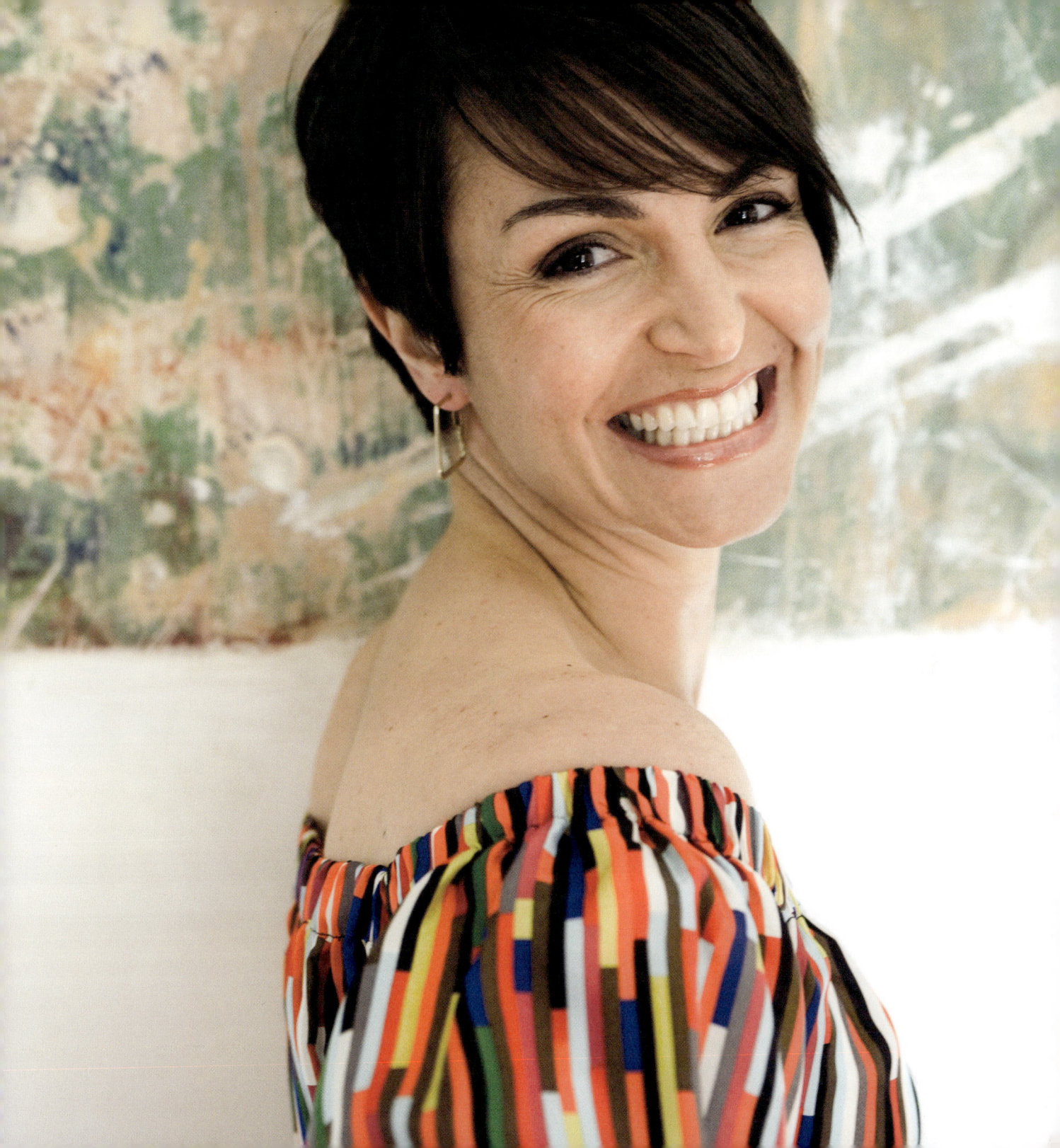

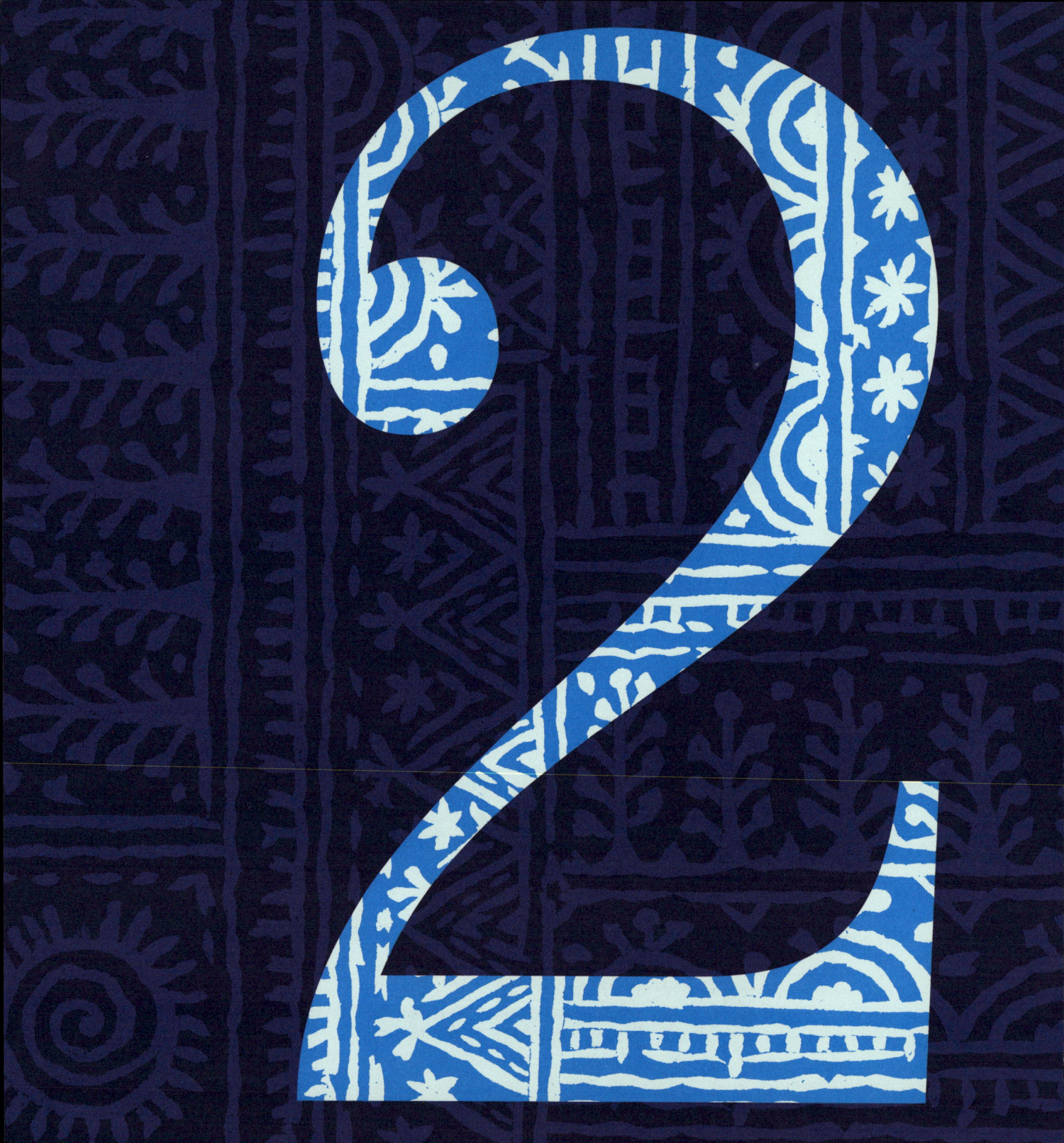

Gain
control

" I try to eat really well most of the time, but sometimes I crave chocolate or something sweet so badly that I can't think about anything else. When I finally give in, I can't stop until I've eaten the whole block. **"**

Carole, 30s, Australian

Have you ever considered why you choose to eat certain foods? So often, diet and health books simply tell us what to eat and why their particular diet is the answer, without actually discussing why we eat in the first place. Perhaps this is why so many of us fail in our attempts to change our diet: we don't understand what drives us to eat. I can talk all day about what to eat, but if you can't control your emotional eating, you won't get anywhere.

To gain some insight into how women feel about food and to gather information about our relationship with food, I carried out a survey. The 72 anonymous responses I received came from a variety of nationalities including Australian, New Zealander, Scottish, Welsh, English, Czech, German, South African and Polish. These women ranged from their 20s to their 70s, and 58 per cent of them said they often ate or drank in response to emotions, with a further 3 per cent admitting they did sometimes. That's pretty much 2 out of 3 of us whose emotions affect what and how we eat.

> " I feel I need to be in the right space to lose weight. If I'm weighed down by emotional issues, it is pointless to try to diet. I need to be in a better situation to start. "
>
> Karen, 50s, Australian

The trouble with this approach is that we will always have tricky emotional times in our lives. We have to learn how to get through these, and everyday emotions, without turning to food for solace. Certainly, if you are having a tough time with some aspect of your life you may lack the energy and headspace to focus on your diet or lifestyle. However, food might be the positive focus you need.

And there is the word—positive. You don't want a weight-oriented focus. You want one that centres on health and vitality.

> ## "Cravings are not really an addiction but a habit."

Sweetie pie

Our food preferences start in the womb. There are fascinating experiments where researchers have taken images of an almost full-term infant in the womb to gauge their reaction to different tastes. When the mother is fed glucose, the sugar is quickly taken into her bloodstream and subsequently crosses the placenta. The resultant images clearly show the infant swallowing more quickly and even smiling in response to the sweet taste. In contrast, when a bitter taste is simulated their look of dislike is unmistakeable and the little mouth closes as if to refuse the food. Those of us who have spent any time with young children know that these food preferences continue into childhood, hence the ubiquitous battle to 'eat your veggies' (because they have a slightly bitter taste) and prevent overindulgence on sweet treats.

These food preferences are in part an evolutionary survival mechanism. In nature sweet foods are usually safe and contain valuable carbohydrates our bodies require. Bitter foods, on the other hand, could be poisonous and we would have had to rely on experienced elders to guide us to plants that could safely be eaten. The foods available to us in the past were whole natural foods, making it practically impossible to overeat and get fat. To survive we would have had to renounce those simple childhood tastes pretty quickly.

Today's world is different. A vast array of sweeter 'children's food' can stop them from developing mature adult tastes. The psychology of eating is also involved here. From an early age we are taught that treats are for 'good girls and boys', and it's hard to break this pattern with our own kids. Food is also commonly used to cheer us up—'Never mind, here's an ice cream to make you feel better'. It's little wonder, then, that as adults we seek similar foods to re-enact these learned responses.

Sweet, energy-dense products surround us, making it really hard for us not to indulge. When you read the ingredients list of regular food items in the supermarket you'll be amazed how many products contain sugar, even in savoury foods such as pies, canned vegetables and pasta sauce. By overly stimulating the sweet end of the flavour palate, we seem to skew our food preferences in that direction. The more you eat these foods, the less likely you are to want to eat healthier, wholesome food. You are conditioned to like and crave sweet tastes.

Good taste

It's not just sugary foods that upset our taste buds. Salt is also overused. Eating too much salt can dull your sense of taste. I'm not talking here about a sprinkling on a poached egg. I mean the huge amounts of salt that are used in processed foods, giving you more than could ever be consumed in a natural food diet. The result is that the subtle tastes of fresh food are lost in a sea of flavoured processed food. If you eat these sorts of foods regularly it will undoubtedly affect your satisfaction after eating. Just think of the tag line for a brand of potato chips, 'Once you pop you can't stop'.

Nothing more than cravings

Cravings, whether for sweet or salty treats, are not really an addiction but a habit. If you always have a biscuit with a cup of tea, that's exactly what you will want whenever you sit down with a cup of tea. If you always have a muffin at your local café, the association is hard to break. Popcorn or a choc-top at the movies, a piece of chocolate after dinner ... The list goes on. Whatever the food association is for you, these are simply habits. If they are problematic, that is, if they are holding you back from reaching your goals, you must work on breaking the habits, otherwise nothing will change.

"Eating too much salt can dull your taste buds."

53

The many guises of sugar

A little sugar in an overall healthy food will do no harm, particularly if it makes the food more palatable and makes you more likely to eat it. But avoid products that have sugar added when there is an alternative with none, for example some canned vegetables and sauces. And I prefer items that use the obvious sugars as they tend to be more 'homemade' in style and less likely to have other undesirable additives.

In moderation, if at all

- **Obvious sugars** Brown sugar, raw sugar, caster sugar, granulated sugar, confectioner's sugar, invert sugar.

- **Syrups** Glucose syrup, golden syrup, corn syrup, rice syrup and (probably worst of all) high-fructose corn syrup (HFCS).

- **Molasses** These sugars come from a few steps up in the sugar-refining process. There might be minute levels of minerals from the original plant, but that doesn't make it any healthier than sugar.

- **Words that end in –ose** Sucrose, dextrose, fructose, maltose, galactose, lactose and glucose. These are simple sugars found naturally in foods, but are also refined and added to food products. The effect on health is not always the same. For example, fructose is fruit sugar, but when extracted and added to soft drinks and processed foods, it can crank up the storage of body fat.

- **Words that end in –ol** Maltitol, lactitol, mannitol, sorbitol and xylitol. These are sugar alcohols often used to replace sugar in many 'sugar-free' foods. Though they have fewer kilojoules, they can give you bloating, flatulence and diarrhoea if you're not used to them or you consume them in excess.

- **Artificial sweeteners** Latest studies show that these don't help you to lose weight and we really don't know their effect over a lifetime, particularly at increasingly high levels.

Best natural sugars

- **Fruit juice concentrate** Much better than some of the other sugars because it is closer to nature. But it's still sugar, even with a few of the micronutrients from the fruit still present . I buy fruit spread and biscuits sweetened with fruit juice concentrate for my kids, and I often use apple juice concentrate in my cooking at home.

- **Honey** We've always enjoyed honey—it couldn't be more natural or minimally processed. The pure floral honeys have the lowest GI values. Manuka honey, with a stated UMF (Unique Manuka Factor), has antibacterial properties and so may help to treat certain bacterial infections. The other advantage of honey is that it's very sweet, so a little goes a long way. Use it to sweeten healthy foods such as a drizzle on the top of a steaming bowl of rolled grain porridge, or to sweeten homemade oat cookies or fruit muffins.

- **Maple syrup** Made by concentrating the sap collected from maple trees. It's far less processed than other sugars and syrups, and contains significant levels of several micronutrients. It's also low GI, provided you buy the real thing and not the cheaper imitation maple-flavoured syrups that are made from glucose syrup or some other cheap bulk sweetener, plus flavourings and other undesirable additives. Real maple syrup is not quite as sweet as honey and has a distinctive flavour.

- **Agave nectar/syrup** This comes from the agave plant (a kind of cactus) native to Mexico, where it has been used as a natural sweetener for thousands of years. Minimal processing or heat is involved in its production, retaining many micronutrients. It also has a low GI and can be used instead of sugar in many recipes. It's now widely available in whole food shops and in some major supermarkets. Sammie uses it in her recipe for toasted nut and seed topping (page 160).

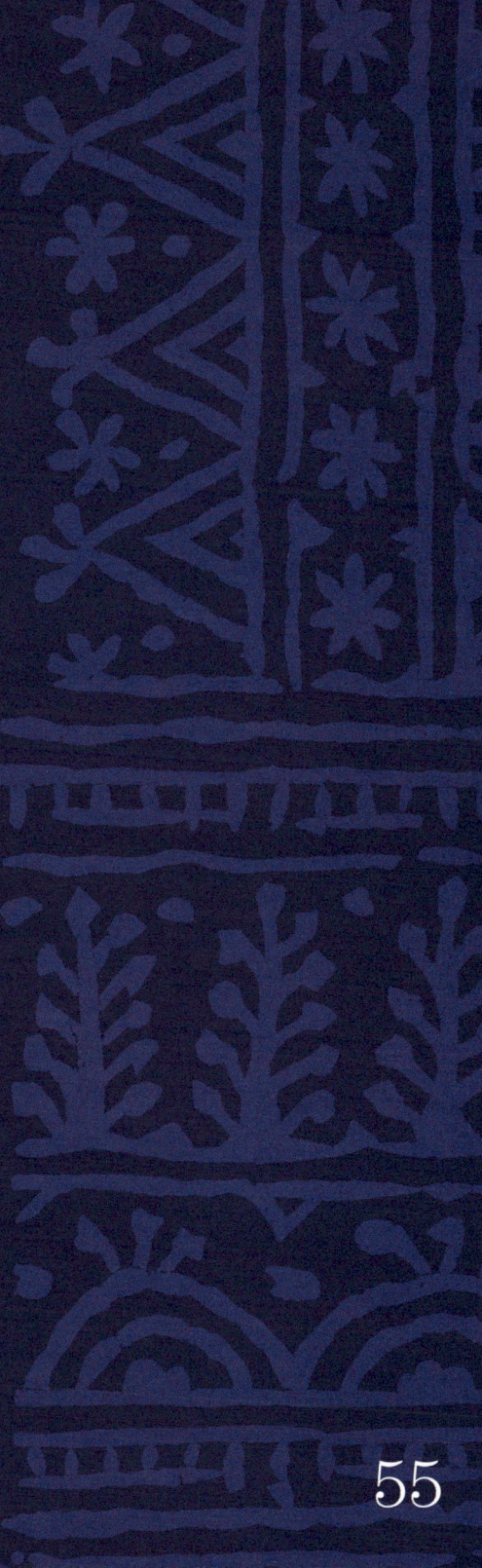

Interestingly Ayurveda, the ancient Hindu health system, teaches something along these lines. A friend and nutrition colleague recently completed a one-month detox with her yoga school. It was based on Ayurvedic principles and the interesting thing to me was the principle for achieving satiation. Ayurveda teaches that all tastes—sweet, sour, salty, bitter, pungent and astringent—must be included in a meal for us to feel satisfied and complete. Every meal in my friend's detox was balanced to include these tastes, while also eliminating certain foods and drinks. The anecdotal reports from those involved were amazingly positive.

While I don't profess to know much about Ayurvedic teachings, this idea of satisfaction from flavours makes sense. We all know the feeling of choosing to eat what we believe is the healthier option, only to crave something else at the end of the meal. We don't need to learn complicated food combinations here, nor am I going to suggest we adopt the Ayurvedic way. But it does tell us that gaining satisfaction from our meals and snacks is crucial in stopping food cravings and emotional eating.

Take a tip from these teachings and try to include different tastes in the same meal. For example, you might combine the pungent taste of spices in an Asian-style curry, along with the slightly bitter taste of stir-fried greens, with a touch of sour lemon juice squeezed over the top, finished with the sourness of natural yoghurt complemented by the sweetness of a fresh fruit salad. You needn't include every taste in each meal. But there should be different tastes, and they should be natural. There are lots of great flavour combinations that will help you in chapter 5 (p. 144).

"So what should we do? Stop eating processed foods that are overly salted, artificially flavoured or excessively sweetened. Return to real food and recondition your body to appreciate all tastes."

TRANS FATS: fats created in an industrial process by adding hydrogen to liquid vegetable oils to make them more solid. They raise 'bad' cholesterol (LDL) levels and reduce 'good' (HDL) cholesterol levels in the body. Trans fats are found mostly in fried foods, biscuits, pastries and takeaways. Avoid any food that lists hydrogenated fat/oil as an ingredient.

Chew on this

The social psychologist Leon Rappoport identifies three eating ideologies in his book *How We Eat*. He calls these 'hedonism', 'nutritionism' and 'spirituality'. I prefer 'pleasure', 'health' and 'ethics'.

Pleasure

Hedonism, Rappoport argues, is the major determinant of what we choose to eat. I call this 'pleasure'. In other words, we choose to eat foods that we like and give us pleasure. This ideology also embraces the social aspects of eating. Food and sharing food is an essential part of being human. Consider any culture the world over and food will be a part of celebrations, get-togethers, family bonding, even death. We've all heard the tale of the intrepid traveller having to eat something they consider revolting, rather than offending their local host. Food is part of our culture, part of our definition of who we are and how we interact with each other.

Health

Rappoport calls his second ideology 'nutritionism', which I call 'health'. Eating to support health is not new. Humankind has long believed in the healing powers of food, and the belief has grown enormously in recent years. But choosing what to eat based on our current knowledge can lead to problems. Advice is constantly changing. The advice to switch to margarine from butter took an about turn with the discovery of trans fats. Suddenly butter was back on the menu—at least until the margarine manufacturers found a way of producing their product without trans fats.

'Nutritionism' also ignores other ideologies. With the focus only on the nutrients that foods contain, it fails to recognise the importance of pleasure in food, the social context of eating with friends and family, or of embracing ethical eating or preserving cultural dishes and traditions surrounding food.

There is a wider concept of health that goes beyond physical requirements. We get more from our food than macronutrients and micronutrients. One of the saddest things I ever heard was when a fitness instructor told me she couldn't wait for the day we wouldn't have to eat and could get all our nutrition in a pill. Boy, does that miss the mark

Pleasure	Health	Ethics
• Served us well in the past	• Driven by modern science	• Embodies religious beliefs
• Includes social aspects of eating	• Ignores other ideologies	• Now also includes ethical eating, vegetarianism, animal welfare, etc.
• Causes problems today because of vast array of energy-dense foods	• Loses sight of bigger picture by focusing on nutrients	
	• Much we still don't know	

" Historically, people have eaten for a great many reasons other than biological necessity. Food is also about pleasure, about community, about family and spirituality, about our relationship to the natural world, and about expressing our identity…Eating has been as much about culture as it has been about biology. "

In Defence of Food by Michael Pollan

59

"I am doing rude things to my body here in Italy, taking in such ghastly amounts of cheese and pasta and wine and chocolate and pizza…I'm not exercising, I'm not eating enough fibre, I'm not taking any vitamins. In my real life I have been known to eat organic goat's milk yoghurt sprinkled with wheat germ for breakfast. My real-life days are long gone… Still, when I look at myself in the mirror of the best pizzeria in Naples, I see a bright-eyed, clear-skinned, happy and healthy face. I haven't seen a face like that on me for a long time." *Eat Pray Love* by Elizabeth Gilbert

Ethics

Rappoport's third ideology is 'spirituality', which I call 'ethics'. In the past this term might have been more apt, but in the modern scientific world (at least in the West) it is viewed as slightly hippy-ish. Yet if we extend this idea to include religious beliefs, vegetarianism and the newer ideas of ethical eating, it becomes an ideology of ethics or morality. For example, when I asked the women in my survey if there were any foods they did not eat, several had moral reasons for their choices. One woman doesn't eat veal or foie gras on the basis of the treatment of animals. Many do not eat pork as defined by their religious beliefs. I also include in here respect for food. I'm not a religious person but to me saying grace before a meal, practised less and less as many of us have turned from religion, was a wonderful expression of respect and thanks for the food in front of us. By contrast, much of today's eating is done on the hoof, rushing from one place to the next, squeezing in a quick meal before a meeting or mindless snacking in front of the TV. It's almost as if by losing our respect for food we have lost respect for ourselves and the powerful effect that eating has on our health.

These three ideologies may seem to be in conflict and indeed they often are — 'I really want that chocolate bar *(pleasure)* but know it isn't good for my weight *(health)* and it's imported from Belgium so there's lots of food miles involved and therefore it's not a good environmental choice *(ethics)*!' But once we are aware of them and give them all equal credence, we can begin to intertwine them to provide a satisfying approach to choosing food. I've described what foods to eat — natural, wholesome, minimally processed — but to truly embrace these three ideologies we also have to go back to attitudes to food, eating behaviours and emotional eating.

C'est très yummy

The so-called French Paradox is that despite seeming to eat loads of unhealthy foods—butter, white bread, cheese, creamy sauces and so on—the French do not have the same problems with obesity and heart disease as countries such as the USA, Australia and the UK. Although some researchers question whether this really is the case, there are some major differences in the way the French eat.

Researchers have looked at all sorts of possible reasons for the French Paradox: genetics, drinking habits, consumption of other protective foods such as salad vegetables, fish and olive oil, to name but a few. But none of these have provided a complete answer. However, at least one study has investigated the paradox, not from a nutritional point of view, but from a psychological point of view.

Paul Rozin, Professor of Psychology at the University of Pennsylvania, and colleagues published a study in 1999 in the journal *Appetite* entitled 'Attitudes to food and the role of food in life'. They investigated the cultural differences to food and eating in four different nations: USA, Japan, Belgium and France. The questions they asked were designed to explore seven key areas:

1 **The degree of consumption of foods modified to be 'healthier'**

2 **Concern for healthiness of food habits of self and others**

3 **The extent of worry about, as opposed to savouring of, food**

4 **The effect of food on health**

5 **The importance of food as a positive force in life**

6 **The tendency to associate foods with nutritional versus culinary contexts**

7 **Satisfaction with the healthiness of own diet**

The two most different countries were the USA and France. The Belgians were pretty close to France, while the Japanese were somewhere between the two. There was no difference between the countries in believing the link between diet and health. There was unanimous agreement that there were strong links between diet and heart disease, obesity, cancer and general good health. But that was where the similarity ended.

American eaters
- bought more low-fat, reduced-salt and other modified foods
- worried more about what they eat and the effects on their health
- were more concerned about family and friends who don't eat well
- placed less importance on food as a positive force in life and took less pleasure from it
- tended to associate foods with nutritional factors rather than culinary but were far less likely to consider themselves healthy eaters

French eaters
- did rate themselves to be healthy eaters
- were much more likely to view food positively
- tended to associate food with culinary rather than nutritional factors
- rated the pleasure of food as extremely important

These results surely show us that our attitude to, and relationship with, food is crucial and plays a vital role in achieving good health. It also illustrates that the tide of 'nutritionism' in the States has not curbed weight issues and chronic disease.

 **In a question asking people to circle the word most different from the other two from 'bread, pasta, sauce' the Americans tended to say 'sauce' since the other two are carbohydrates, while the French tended to circle 'bread' since pasta and sauce clearly go together in a meal. Yet despite this apparent awareness and importance of nutritional factors, the Americans are fatter and have higher rates of chronic diseases with strong nutritional links such as type-2 diabetes and heart disease than the French.**

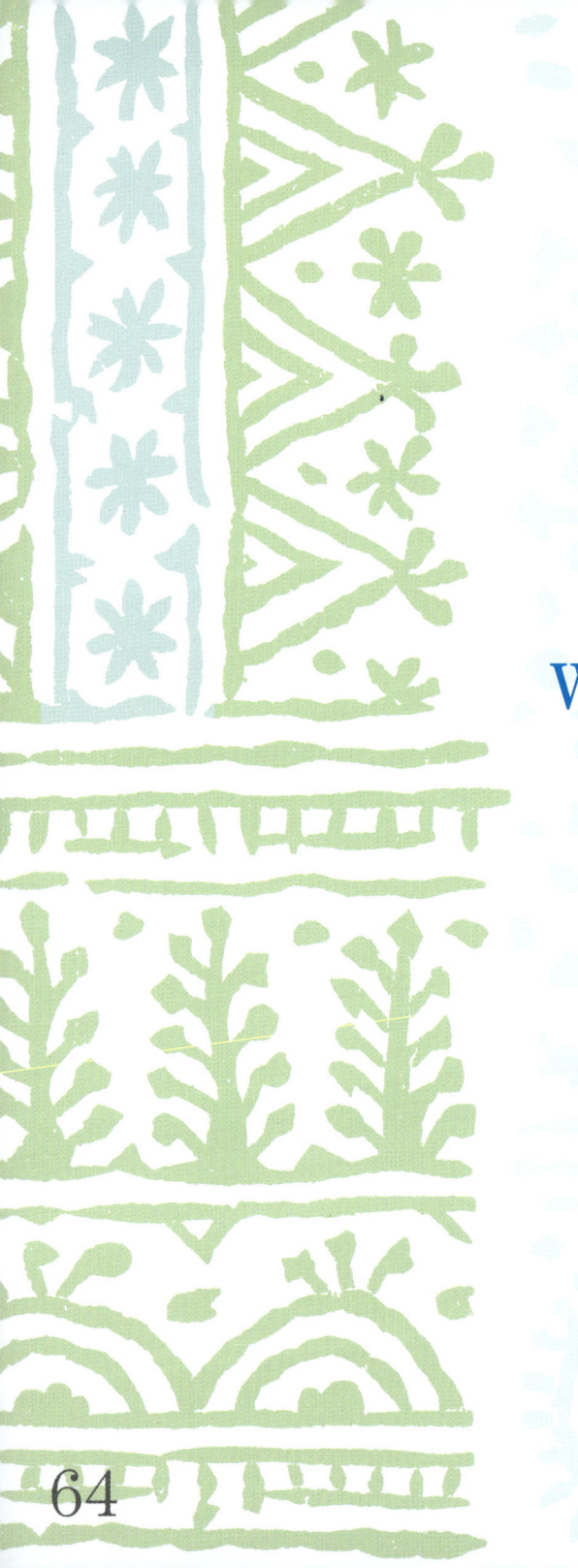

Food quiz

What are your attitudes to food and the role of food in life? Try answering the following questions, taken randomly from the real study.

1 On a scale of 1–4, how much of an effect do you believe diet has on good health?

2 Ice-cream belongs best with: *delicious* or *fattening*?

3 Are the following statements true or false for you:
- Money spent on food is money well spent
- Enjoying food is one of the most important pleasures in my life
- I think about food in a positive, anticipatory way
- I would rather eat my favourite meal than watch my favourite television show
- I am concerned with the health of friends/family who eat poorly

4 Fried egg belongs best with: *breakfast* or *cholesterol*

5 Circle the word that you think is most different from the other two:

bread   pasta   sauce

carbohydrate   bread   butter

I suspect most of us would be like women around the world and rate highly the effect of diet on good health. But how did you fare on the other questions? If you put 'ice-cream' with 'fattening', answered false to the first four statements and true to the last, put 'fried egg' with 'cholesterol' and circled the different words to be 'sauce' and 'butter' you probably share the American attitude to food. A little more French attitude might help you to reach your goals!

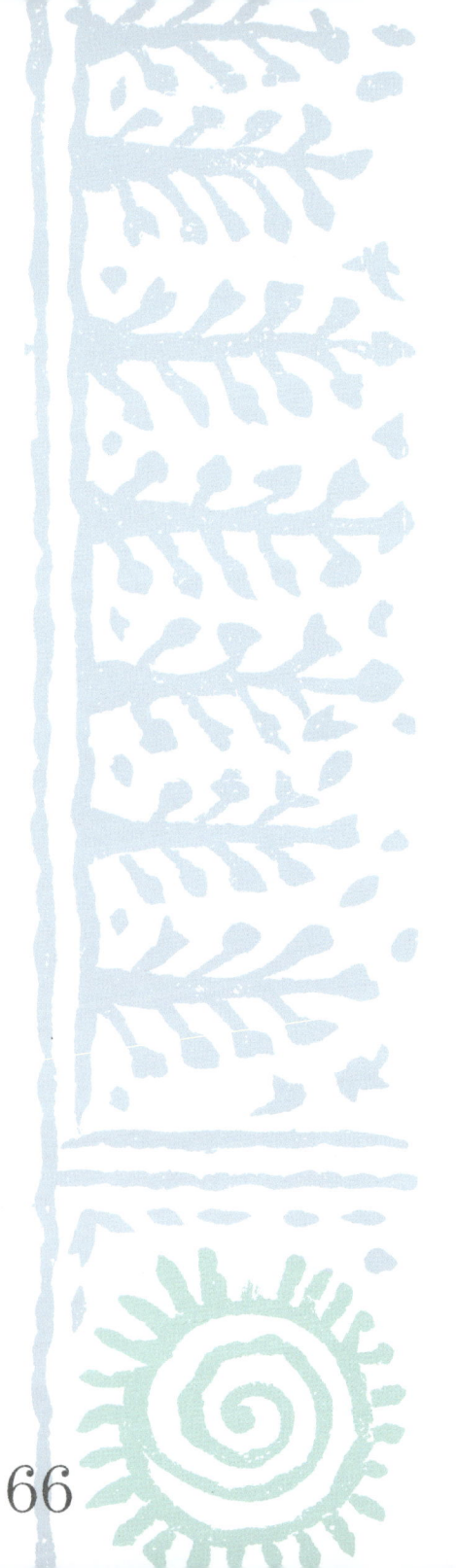

Take your cue

- Do you listen to your body or your environment?
- Do you think about how you eat: what triggers you to start and stop eating?
- Do you start to think about eating when you feel hunger pangs?
- Do you go and get lunch because the clock says it's lunchtime?
- Do you suddenly feel like a snack because the person next to you is having one?
- Do you stop eating when you are satisfied or simply when you've finished everything on your plate?

The responses to these questions relate to two different types of cues to eat and stop eating: internal and external. Internal cues are listening to your own body—you look for food when you are hungry and stop eating when you are full or satisfied. External cues are all the things outside your body that influence your eating.

'In company I sometimes eat a bigger amount than I know I need, especially as I was brought up to eat all the food on my plate—it's difficult to go against such training.' Jane, 60s, UK

This comment demonstrates how an external cue has a big effect on the amount someone eats. Most of us were probably brought up with the same etiquette rules—there are starving children in Ethiopia after all! This is something I have tried to change in raising my own children. Certainly, they often need encouragement to eat but the rule in our house is that they must taste everything on their plate, rather than finish the plate. My hope is that I can nurture their natural ability to control how much they need to eat (an internal cue) rather than become too responsive to external cues. For adults already 'trained' in this way it takes conscious and sustained effort to change the way of thinking.

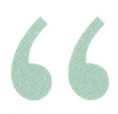

When it comes to controlling appetite and eating we should listen to our bodies and be less influenced by our environment and those around us.

Here are some tips for learning to listen to internal cues:

• Always sit at the table to eat and avoid eating on the run. Make eating conscious not automatic.
• Slow down and put your cutlery down between mouthfuls.
• Turn off the TV.
• Make mealtimes pleasant. Avoid arguing with your partner over dinner.
• Stop eating when satisfied, not full. Try the Okinawans' 80 per cent rule.
• Before you eat, think about how hungry you are. Ask yourself if you are seeking food to fulfil some other need.

Going back to the French and the Americans for a moment, a study published in 2007 shed further light on the differences between the two when it comes to food and eating. Food behaviour expert, Professor Brian Wansink from the Food and Brand Lab at Cornell University, USA, headed an experiment to compare the cues to eating and stopping eating in two groups of students from Paris and Chicago. They had to rate their agreement with statements related to internal cues (for example, 'I usually stop eating when I start to feel full') and external cues (for example, 'I usually stop eating when I've eaten what most think is normal'). You will by now have guessed that the French seemed to be much better at listening to internal cues and were less influenced by the external, environmental cues. When they separated the students by their weight not their nationality, the overweight students tended to respond to external cues far more than the normal weight students. The message is clear—when it comes to controlling appetite and eating we should listen to our bodies and be less influenced by our environment and those around us.

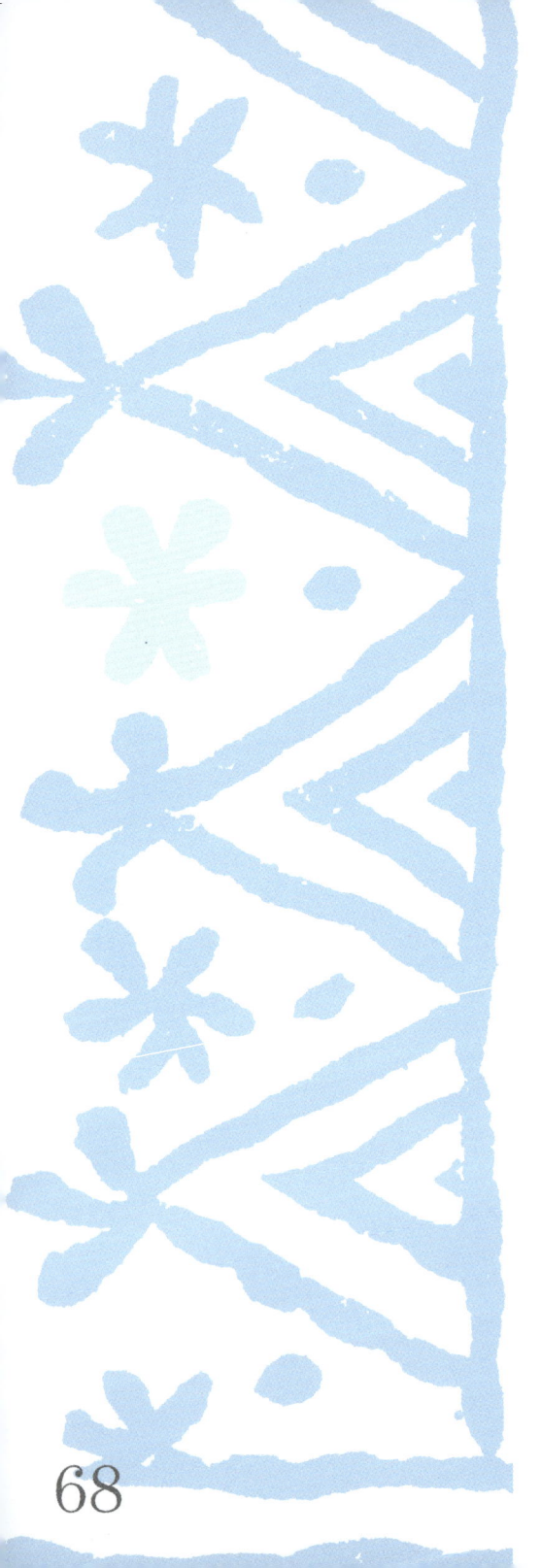

Control freak

I used to have a regular girls-only lunch with friends for a catch-up. One of the girls started to bring a friend and, from the first meeting, it was clear that she had a difficult relationship with food. While the rest of us enjoyed at least two courses, she would order a plate of steamed vegetables, saying, 'I ate earlier' or 'I'm not all that hungry'. She wouldn't have a glass of wine, instead drinking several coffees over the course of lunch. While the rest of us shared our food, tasting all the dishes, she would push the vegetables around the plate and usually give up long before they were finished. She was very slim but I suspect she was at one end of the dietary restraint scale.

Yet it seems that those who are very controlled and restrained in how they eat are more susceptible to falling off the perch when a trigger comes along that breaks their strict control. An emotional upset or simply succumbing to a 'forbidden' food can lead to a dramatic swing towards a total lack of inhibition. It's the classic 'I've blown my diet for today so I may as well eat whatever I want for the rest of the day and start again tomorrow'. Of course, if you have no control and always eat in a uninhibited way you are also likely to have trouble controlling your weight. Most of us are somewhere between the two. The closer you get to either end, the more likely problems will result.

'I had a flatmate who was so vague and out of it we all thought she was really dumb. It turns out she had an eating disorder. She confided in me after I asked her why the fridge was empty! Seriously, she would get up in the middle of the night when we were asleep and eat everything out of the fridge, and then try to get up earlier than us to go and replace it at the supermarket before we noticed … She was so vague because she was always hungry … She ended up going to Overeaters Anonymous four nights a week but still couldn't really control it.' Catriona, 20s, Australian

While this is extreme, many women in my survey described some kind of secretive eating, or confessed that they often eat more when alone than with others. In fact 46 per cent of the women said that they ate differently when alone (not all said they ate more, but in general they said they ate less well). Here are just a few examples:

'I definitely eat more on my own. I wouldn't eat a family block of Cadbury's with people around.' Jackie, 30s, British

'Tend to eat bad things when alone so that no one sees and they don't get disappointed with me.' Kelly, 20s, Australian

'I convince myself that it is OK to sneak in the odd treat as no one knows ... Interesting philosophy—it's like I hide it.' Susan, 30s, British

'Binge eat on ice cream when alone.' Carla, 30s, Australian

'Snack furtively even when I'm alone in the house and no one will ever know.' Mary, 50s, British

'When I am alone, I often eat in a more uncontrolled way.' Anne, 20s, Swiss

A healthier approach for our lunch companion would have been to order a starter and main as we had (or order two starters) but to have made healthy choices that she knew she would also enjoy. By stopping when satisfied, not when the plate was clean, she would have avoided overeating but gained the great enjoyment and appreciation of a delicious meal eaten in good company.

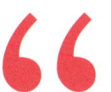

Get the balance right.

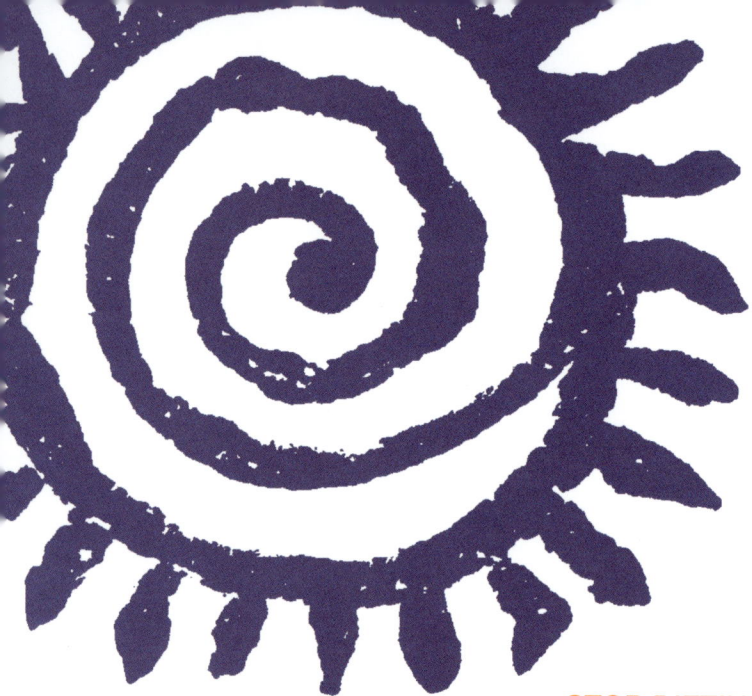

STOP DIETING

If you feel out of control with your eating and succumb to bouts of overeating followed by restraint and dieting, it will take some time to alter your pattern of thinking. The first step in breaking the cycle is to stop dieting. Even the thought of going on a diet is enough to send some into a bingeing session. A study published in the *Journal of Abnormal Psychology* (Urbszat, D., 2002) looked at this phenomenon. They took a group of women known to be either restrained or unrestrained eaters, and told half of them that they were assigned to the 'diet group', which would commence tomorrow. They then gave all the women a taste-rating task and measured their subsequent food consumption. The unrestrained eaters ate the same amount of food, regardless of whether they thought they would be dieting the next day or not. The restrained eaters, however, ate significantly more (more than double) if they believed they were going on a diet than those who were not. It seems that even planning to go on a diet can trigger overeating in women who are restrained eaters.

STOP FEELING GUILTY ABOUT FOOD

'I still think about food too much. I look at others and wish I could eat in a more relaxed way. If cakes are at work and I have one, I go home and overeat thinking I have already ruined things by having a fattening cake! Crazy.' Jill, 40s, British

70

> **It's what happens regularly over time that really counts. No one food, one meal or even one whole day of eating badly is going to do much damage.**

Only 17 per cent of women in my survey said they never felt guilty over what or how much they had eaten, so this is something that affects the vast majority of us. Eleven per cent of the women confessed that they had actually made themselves sick due to these guilty feelings. One woman who had struggled with bulimia when she was younger confessed to having an ongoing battle with food.

Feeling guilt over what is done is pointless. No one food, one meal or even one whole day of eating badly is going to do much damage. It's what happens regularly over time that really counts. You might eat too much chocolate cake at a birthday party and feel fat the next morning. But if we could really measure your body fat levels there would be no discernible difference. However, if you ate chocolate cake every night for a week then we would start to see a difference. Feeling guilty over eating is such a negative emotion that it cannot help build a positive relationship to food. What is done is done, so move on. A more effective approach is to say, 'OK, I've enjoyed a large meal and that chocolate cake was delicious. I'll go for an extra-long walk tomorrow and make sure I get back on track with my usual healthy meals.'

Hunger–Satiation Rating Scale

1. Absolutely ravenous—you will eat anything and will tend to overeat
2. Ravenous—you can't think of anything but finding food
3. Hungry—your stomach's rumbling and you're ready to eat
4. Slightly hungry—you're thinking about food but could wait longer
5. Neutral—you don't feel particularly hungry but could eat if food was offered
6. Not quite satisfied—you've eaten a little food but not enough to satisfy
7. Satisfied—you feel you have eaten enough but could eat more
8. Eighty per cent full—you're completely satisfied but not completely full
9. Uncomfortably full—you have eaten a little too much
10. Absolutely stuffed—you've overeaten to the point where you feel a bit sick and need to lie down!

LISTEN TO YOUR BODY

So many of us have become so accustomed to the 'noise' of life that we forget to listen to ourselves. We all sometimes eat for reasons other than hunger—boredom, being upset, to cheer ourselves up, to give us energy, to treat ourselves—and that is perfectly normal. It only becomes problematic when the external cues take dominance over the internal ones (like the American and French study example mentioned previously). Dietitians often have their clients keep a food-awareness diary where you record not only what and when you eat, but also how you feel before you eat and how hungry you are. The Hunger–Satiation Scale on this page is useful in helping you to identify your reasons for eating. For example, do you really want food or would something else actually fulfil your need better? If you find that you do overeat, this scale helps identify why it's happening. Do you overeat because you tend to skip meals and allow yourself to get over hungry? Or do you overeat in response to a particular emotion? Or perhaps you overeat in certain situations, such as in a favourite restaurant or with a particular group of friends.

 You are in control

The Australian GP and eating behaviour expert Dr Rick Kausman recommends in his excellent book *If not dieting then what?* that before eating you ask yourself, 'I can have it if I really want it, but do I really feel like it?' This embraces exactly my perspective. You are in control of what you eat. You are not on a diet and you don't have to feel deprived of foods you want and like. But do you really feel like the food at this moment? Often you'll discover that the impulse passes or that in fact you are just angry, frustrated or upset and this would be better managed by phoning a friend or going for a walk to calm down. It also helps to break the habit cycle. Earlier I mentioned always having a biscuit with a cup of tea— but do you really feel like the biscuit or are you having one simply because it's there and you always do so?

The second part of listening to your body relates to when to stop eating: learn to recognise when you are satisfied (about a rating of 6 on the Hunger–Satiation Scale) and don't eat until you are uncomfortably full. Behaviours including always sitting at the table to eat (which prevents mindless eating in front of the TV, for example), avoiding doing anything else while eating (except talking when in company of course!) and slowing down the pace of eating, will help you take control of this. So many of us wolf our food down in order to get onto the next thing. This makes it practically impossible for your body to react with satiety cues to the brain that reduce your appetite and 'tell' you when to stop—you're already overfull before it has had a chance! Some people also find it helpful to practise leaving something on their plate to break the habit of cleaning it completely. Do whatever works to help you listen more to the internal body cues.

of what you eat. "

FEEL GOOD ABOUT YOURSELF

Try to find non-food means of dealing with emotions. You may have noticed that you tend to eat better when you feel good about yourself and are generally happy about life. It's when we're tired, depressed, angry or not feeling attractive that we tend towards an unhealthier diet.

I asked the women in my survey if they ate in response to everyday emotions: 58 per cent said they did, with a further 3 per cent agreeing that they did sometimes. Since more than half of these women were not overweight, this shows us that this is not necessarily a problem, at least for weight control (although for many women still in their 20s and 30s this may catch up with them later). In fact, in a way it shows the power of food and its ability to affect our emotions.

'I definitely believe that eating badly or too much is connected to emotions. When I was younger I didn't like myself and found comfort in eating chocolate and cakes. As a result I reached a size 16. When I was happy and confident I ate less.' Ruth, 30s, British

Emotional rescue

I asked women about what food and drinks they reached for in response to four emotions.

TOP 3 FOODS AND DRINKS CONSUMED IN RESPONSE TO

ANGER	SADNESS	STRESS	JOY
Alcohol 38%	Chocolate 29%	Alcohol 40%	Champagne 45%
Pasta and starchy foods 10%	Alcohol 24%	Sweet foods 24%	Celebratory cakes 10%
Sweet foods 10%	Sweet foods 14%	Junk and fatty foods 14%	Healthy food 5%
Chocolates 10%			Chocolate 5%
Fatty foods (primarily chips or cheese) 7%			

The three negative emotions had distinctly different patterns to the positive emotion of joy. Barring the celebratory champagne, about a third of the women (who confessed to sometimes eating or drinking in response to emotions) did not eat or drink when joyful. If they did, it was with cake or other foods associated with a social or celebratory occasion, rather than a food they sought out or craved. This was also the only emotion to which any woman reported selecting healthy foods. Clearly most of us eat better when we're happy.

Alcohol featured prominently in response to all emotions, but particularly in response to anger and stress. I'm sure many of you can relate to getting home after a stressful day and pouring a glass of wine or a G&T. I'm not about to tell you that's wrong, because relaxing with a drink can indeed help. But it does become a major risk to health when you are repeatedly stressed or angry and this is your only outlet. Regular drinking pushes you over the healthy limits for women. Not only does it become a real threat to your health, it also starts affecting the way you look and feel. Since alcohol also lowers inhibitions, you often lose your resolve to eat well and you're more likely to ring for takeaway than cook a healthy meal.

Chocolate stood out as a response to being upset and this ties in with the childhood conditioning to 'cheer yourself up' with a treat food. Chocolate also releases 'feel-good' hormones such as serotonin, but they are not the only food to do this. It seems that the pleasure and comforting aspect of chocolate is the real key. Sweet foods were also a popular response to being upset, but even more so to stress. This may be linked to the hormonal response to stress—the classic 'fight or flight' reaction. Stress hormones are essentially getting the body ready for a flurry of activity—fighting the threat or running from it. It makes sense that we should crave sugar in such an event to provide the immediate, fast energy our body needs in such a scenario. Unfortunately, our bodies haven't quite caught up with modern life where stress does not result in activity. In fact, for those with desk jobs it probably means just the opposite—more time at the desk to work out the problem.

> ## If you feel confident about how you look, you'll cope better with the day, you'll feel happier, have more energy and therefore be more active—which all leads to better eating.

So what's the solution?

We can't always be contented so that we'll eat better. But we can do our best to have respect for ourselves and make an effort to improve how we feel about ourselves. Think about how much better you feel when you've had a shower, put on a little make-up, styled your hair and pull on a nice outfit. This might sound really shallow, and I'm not suggesting we have to be polished and dressed up every day, but consider how you feel at the opposite end of the spectrum—unwashed hair, no make-up, wearing a pair of stretched, unflattering trackies. It does make a difference to what and how you eat.

But don't go along the lines of 'I'll buy myself something nice to wear once I've lost weight', even if you have a lot of weight to lose. You'll never get there if you don't feel good along the way. One of the best pieces of advice I received about coping with a new baby before my first child arrived was to have a shower and get dressed as soon as possible in the morning. It's the same principle. If you feel confident about how you look, you'll cope better with the day, you'll feel happier, have more energy and therefore be more active—which all leads to better eating. You don't need an expensive wardrobe. What you do to feel good is up to you. For some it might simply be a well-fitted pair of trackies and a matching fitted T-shirt, a slick of mascara and lipgloss and a comb through the hair. Your 'look' has to be practical and reflective of what you do during the day. Whether you're a mum at home with young kids or a corporate highflier, the point is to feel good about yourself.

Dealing with emotions in ways that don't involve food and drink takes more time. Try to express those emotions and write them down. Psychologists advise you to identify the emotion first, think it through and recognise why you are feeling the way you are. Then try to come up with a healthy outlet for the emotion. If you come home from work incredibly tense and stressed, try putting on your trainers and heading out the door for a brisk walk before you reach for the glass of chardy. By the time you get back, have a shower and change, you'll have released some of that tension and will be less likely to over-drink. If you are angry and upset, perhaps at your partner, rather than delving into the biscuit box to cheer yourself up, phone a friend and talk through the issue first. We could come up with loads of scenarios but the bottom line is to find an outlet for the emotion that doesn't involve food.

WATCH YOUR MOUTH

Be aware of destructive eating behaviours. Try to intervene decisively before they take hold.

• Don't eat while driving, walking down the street or directly from the fridge or pantry. You can't possibly appreciate your food and are likely to over-eat, get indigestion—or worse, crash the car!

• If you're a mum to a toddler, don't finish their plate, nibble on their bits and pieces while preparing their meal and then eat your own meal later. It feels like you ate nothing but it all adds up.

• Make an effort not to snack in front of the TV or at the movies. Mindless eating means that you're not really enjoying your food and you'll eat far more than you realise.

Eight great strategies to reduce emotional and binge eating

1 Give your eating some structure—three meals plus one or two snacks a day

2 No skipping meals—you'll just overeat later

3 Try not to go more than four hours without food—becoming really hungry can trigger a binge

4 Don't ban any food or drink—labelling foods as 'forbidden' only makes you want them more

* **If you feel your emotional eating is serious and you regularly end up bingeing and feeling out of control, consider seeing a professional therapist. It sounds very 'LA' but it might just be the help you need to start changing your relationship with food.**

5 Stop obsessing over the fat, carbs or protein in food—choose wholesome, natural foods you know make you feel good

6 Allow yourself treat foods in small but regular quantities—as you realise that you can have them whenever you want, you'll probably find you don't want them as much as you thought you would

7 Look for other means of dealing with your emotions—move out of your comfort zone and try something new like meditation, yoga, or learning relaxation techniques

8 Surround yourself with people who influence your eating and lifestyle in a positive and healthy way

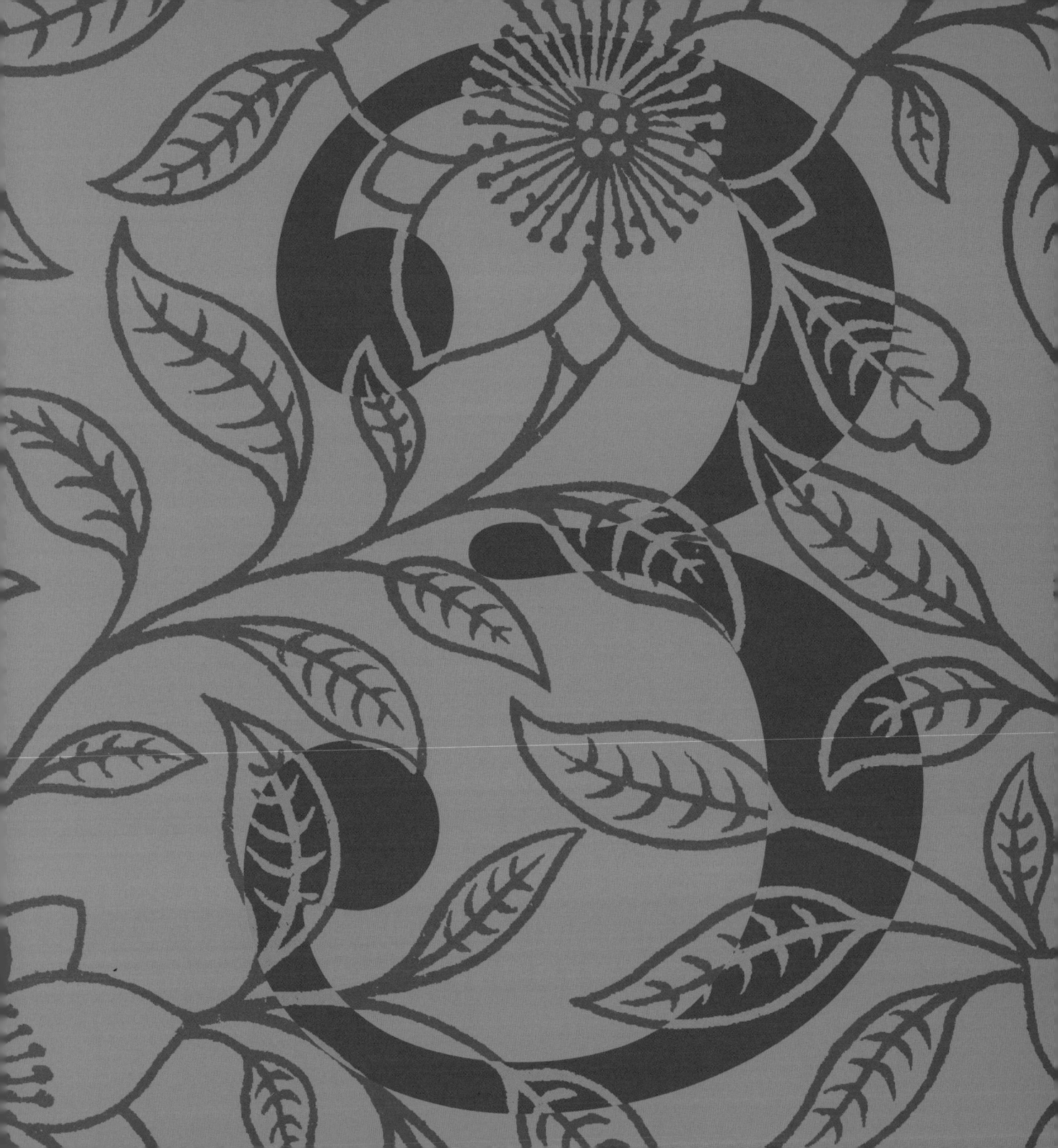

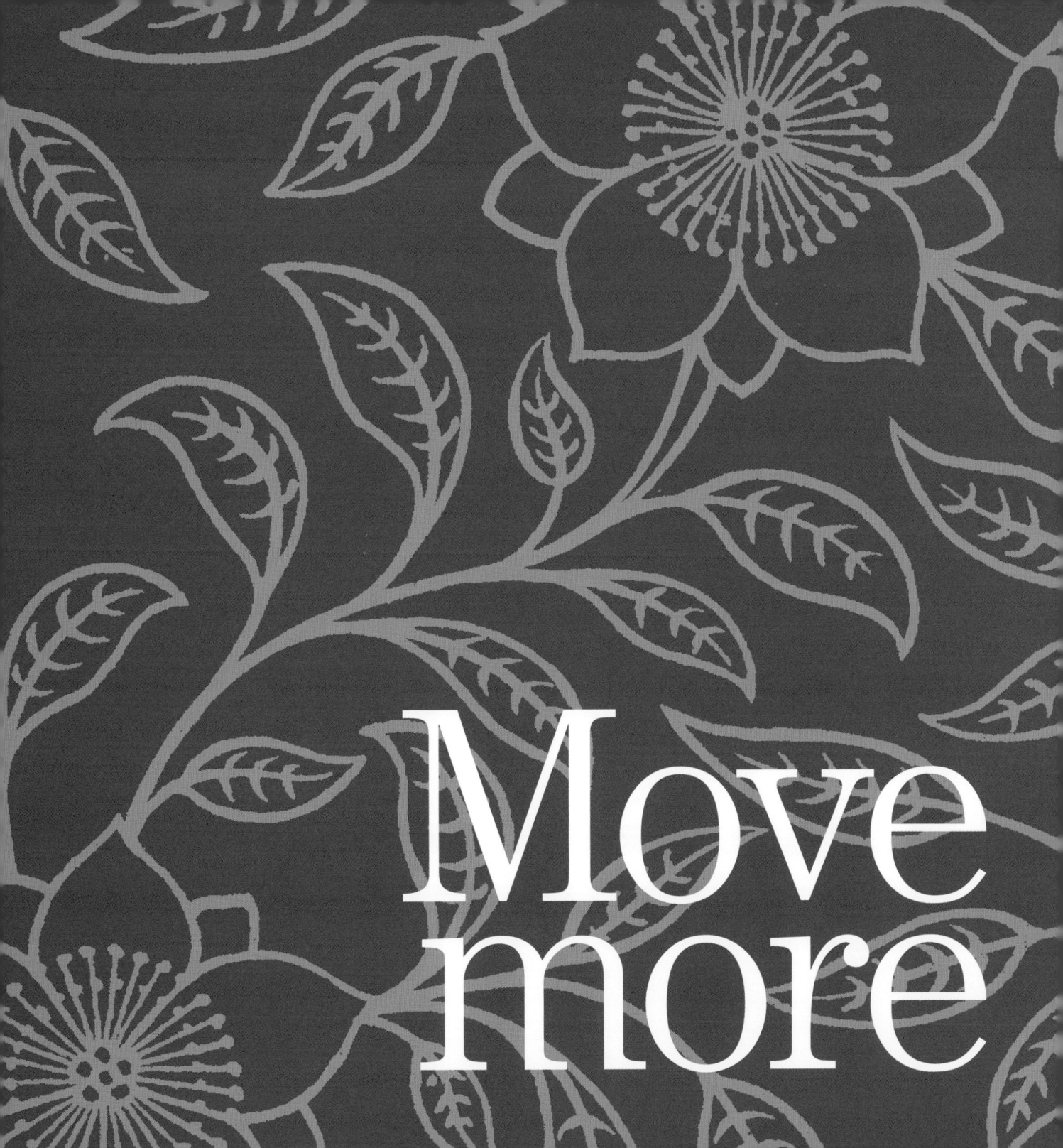

Move
more

"Being fit should be your main priority over weight control."

We all know that exercise is good for the heart and lungs, and we know it's essential to reduce our long-term risk of a number of diseases. But these motivations are too far removed from our daily lives to help most of us get out of bed for an early morning run, or make it to the gym after work, or find the time to get to our yoga class. If you ask women who exercise regularly why they do it, they inevitably say, 'Because it makes me feel and look good'. It's not just about weight control either. Those who are slim but do no exercise are often worse off in various health measurements than those who are fat but fit. As it happens, a lot of evidence points to the fact that being fit should be your main priority over weight control. Besides, if you get moving, chances are you'll find your body changing shape without you consciously thinking about it. My advice is don't make weight loss the only measurable outcome.

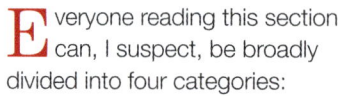

"The great thing about doing lots of exercise is that you can afford to eat more while still maintaining your weight—hurray!"

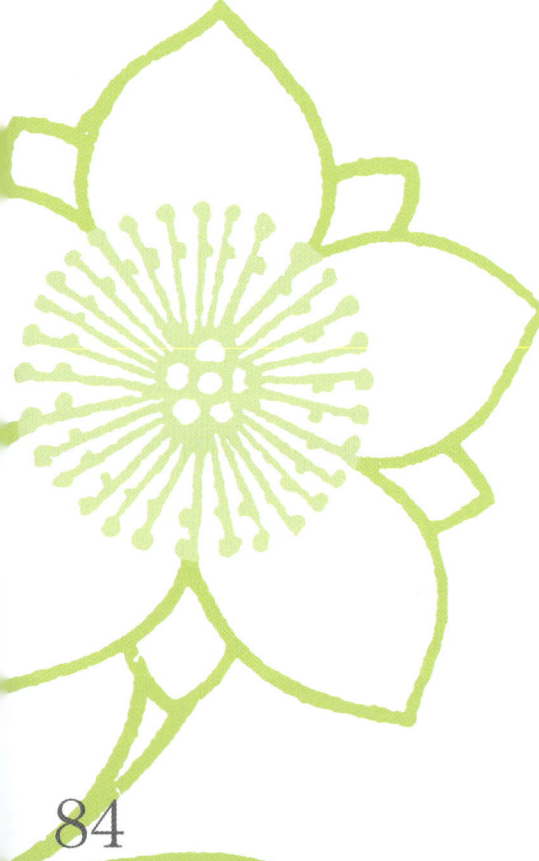

Everyone reading this section can, I suspect, be broadly divided into four categories:

A Regular exercisers who are looking for new ideas, or confirmation that you are exercising in the most effective ways.

B Exercise flirts who alternate between bouts of activity and being sedentary, who are looking for ways to make exercise more regular.

C Novice exercisers who don't know where or how to begin and are scared of failing.

D Naturally slim women who, with no weight control to worry about, find it difficult to drum up the motivation to exercise.

Regardless of weight, age, lifestyle, family history or star sign, we all need to exercise. So, if you are woman (a), fantastic! Keep up the good work. I hope you find something of value in this section. But this is really written for those of you who fall into the categories (b), (c) or (d). You are in the majority, and moving more is the only way you can achieve your potential to look and feel your absolute best.

The great thing about doing lots of exercise is that you can afford to eat more while maintaining your weight—hurray! This is the way it's supposed to be. If we exercise routinely, we can eat the amount of food we are programmed to eat instead of constantly fighting our bodies to get used to smaller amounts of food. This in turn makes it much easier to get all the nutrients our bodies need without resorting to supplements. The less food you eat, the harder it is to meet the daily requirements for all micronutrients. The other great thing about doing more exercise is that our bodies get even better at balancing energy, making weight control easier.

Good reasons to get moving

Fat or thin, here are some of the benefits of making exercise a regular part of your life. The right exercise can:

- give you more energy
- give you shapely shoulders so you can carry off a strappy summer dress
- improve your skin
- sculpt your bum so you look great in your favourite jeans
- improve your concentration and attention span
- improve your strength and balance so everyday tasks are easier

- stop you from ever getting constipated again
- allow you to eat more, but also make you feel like eating good food more often
- slow the ageing process
- make you burn more fat all the time, making long-term weight control much easier
- help you sleep better
- strengthen your immune system so you catch fewer colds and flu

So how much exercise should you do and what sort?

Activity versus exercise—at a glance

Activity All the little acts of movement we perform over the course of the day. Includes walking to work or walking the dog, cleaning the house, picking up after the kids, gardening, ironing, sex (although this could be exercise depending on intensity and duration!), standing in the queue at the bank, climbing the stairs and so on.

Exercise The more formal sessions of usually more intense movement. More structured for the desired result. Includes going for a run/swim/cycle, tennis, taking part in a team sport, doing a yoga/group fitness/dance/Pilates class, or taking part in a water sport such as rowing or kayaking.

It's good to separate activity from exercise because many people make the mistake of thinking only about exercise. They follow the mandatory 'three times a week' rule and wonder why they are struggling to reach their goals. The thing is that even if you work really hard in three hour-long exercise sessions, that still leaves 165 hours in the week where you are more than likely almost completely sedentary. To give us a more realistic idea of how much exercise and activity we should be doing, let's ask ourselves, 'What would Paleolithic woman do?'

Born to be active

Women (and men) were far more active in the past than we are today. Their daily life involved walking, running, climbing, carrying loads, lifting, stretching and jumping. Exercise was an everyday part of getting food, keeping safe and ultimately surviving. One of the other main differences from how we live today was that the level of activity, or the amount of food eaten, was not constant. There were cycles of activity and rest, feast and famine.

Far too many of us are stuck in a feast and rest cycle.

That was then, this is now

Today, we have similar amounts of food from day to day but only small changes in our energy output through exercise. And we don't get close to the levels of exercise of our ancestors. Far too many of us are stuck in a feast and rest cycle and we completely bypass famine and activity. In other words, there's little opportunity to empty the fuel tanks yet we continue to take more and more fuel on board.

We don't need to go as far back as the hunter–gatherers to see this dramatic difference in energy outputs. Go back a mere two or three generations and the differences are stark. In an attempt to illustrate this, the Australian public health expert Professor Garry Egger, along with colleagues from Maastrict University in the Netherlands, conducted an experiment comparing the energy demands of modern sedentary office workers and the early Australian settlers of 150 years ago. Seven men simulated the lives of the settlers by living in Old Sydney Town, an historical theme park near Sydney, based on life around the early 1900s. The volunteers had to avoid all modern technology as much as possible and wore a sophisticated device to measure their activity levels. A second group of seven men with typically sedentary modern jobs continued with their normal routine, also wearing the activity-monitoring device. Both groups were monitored for a week.

The men in the historical group were on average 1.6 times more active than the modern men—in walking terms that's equivalent to walking an extra 8 kilometres a day. In fact, the two 'historical' men who adhered most closely to the 'settler' way of live had even greater activity levels—2.3 times those of the modern men, or the equivalent of walking an extra 16 kilometres a day (Egger, G. et al 2001).

This is only a simulation and used a small number of men, yet the results are in line with other estimates of activity level change. Consider the effect on energy balance (and weight control) over the course of a year if you were to walk 16 kilometres every day on top of your normal routine. For a 60 kilogram woman walking at a brisk pace it would take over three hours to cover 16 kilometres and she would burn off roughly 2700 kilojoules (645 calories). Over the course of a year the difference in energy expenditure between the modern-day woman and her active ancestor is 985,500 kilojoules, or the equivalent of 26.6 kilograms in body fat!

So, you're thinking that's all very well, but who on earth has the time or the inclination to fit in three hours of walking a day? The common advice to exercise for 30 minutes three times a week is nowhere near enough to really influence weight control. It may provide a few health benefits, and certainly some is better than none, but if you want the best results, think about how active you are now and how much more you could do. To get even close to these levels of activity you have to think not just about how much exercise you fit into your week, but how active you are from day to day.

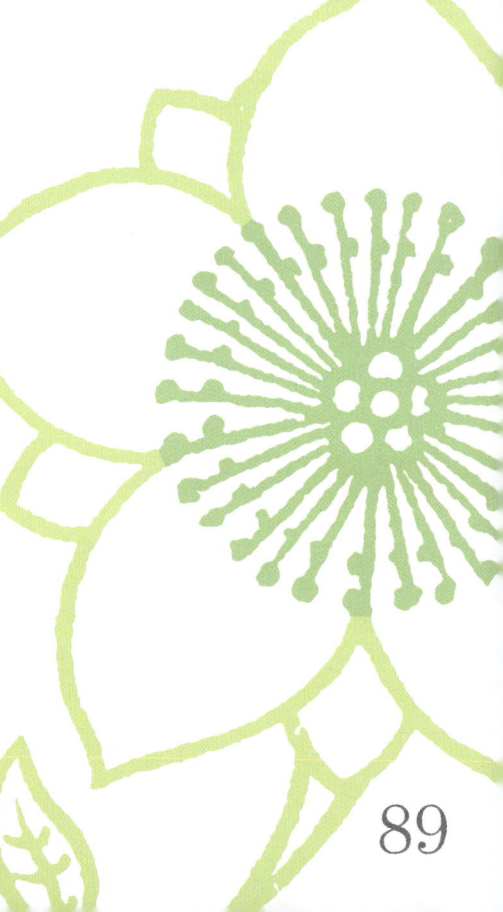

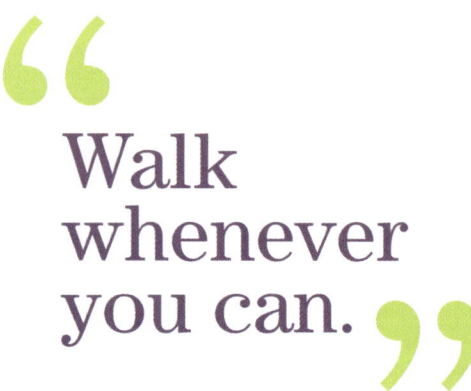

> **Walk whenever you can.**

Walk the walk—the benefits

Sure—we can't devote three hours every day to walking, but if you added just 10 minutes of brisk walking every day for the next year, you could burn an extra 1.4 kilograms of fat. That's enough to prevent the usual age-related weight gain that occurs insidiously, without us even realising it until several years and several extra kilos down the track. And if you walk more, the potential benefits only increase.

Walking is such a basic activity that I always give it the utmost priority. Regardless of whatever other activity and exercise you do in the week, walk whenever you can. This is the cornerstone to being more active in your daily life.

Walk off the weight	
Walk for this many minutes every day ...	**... And you could burn this much fat over the next year**
10	1.4 kg
20	2.8 kg
30	4.1 kg
40	5.5 kg
50	6.9 kg
60	8.3 kg

Note: Figures are based on a 60 kg woman. If you weigh more you will burn more energy and vice versa.

8 great reasons to walk

1   (Almost) anyone can do it

2   No special equipment is required, except for a comfortable pair of shoes

3   You can fit it into your usual schedule by accumulating minutes of walking across the day

4   It doesn't cost a cent

5   It's a great stress reliever

6   It's highly conducive to brainstorming (some of my best ideas have come to me during my walk)

7   You can do it on your own, with a friend, as a group, or pushing a pram or wheelchair

8   You can do it at any suitable time—morning, noon or night!

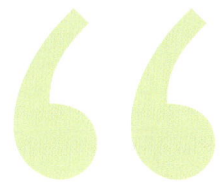

You have to think about how active you are from day to day.

How much is enough?

There's still disagreement among scientific experts as to exactly how much exercise and activity we need to do for optimal health. The International Association for the Study of Obesity (IASO) came to their consensus by again comparing modern activity levels with our ancestors. Our hunter–gatherer sisters ate more, but they also did more exercise, so that roughly a third of the kilojoules from their food was 'spent' on exercise. Today we eat less, but we also exercise considerably less, spending only a seventh of the kilojoules from our food on exercise.

IASO recommends increasing our exercise energy output to match the ratio of our distant relatives—in other words we should aim to expend a third of our daily kilojoule intake on exercise. We can take an average woman weighing 60 kilograms as an example. She consumes about 8000 kilojoules a day. To spend a third of this on exercise she has to burn 2670 kilojoules. She currently burns about 1120 kilojoules (a seventh of her intake) so she has to burn an extra 1550 kilojoules to meet the challenge. How could she do it? Let's look at the time she would have to spend on various forms of exercise or activity to meet this goal.

1 calorie = 4.2 kilojoules

To convert kilojoules to calories, divide by 4.2

Burning up

How much time does it take a 60 kg woman to burn an extra 1550kJ?

- 120 minutes of general housework

- 90 minutes of general gardening

- 70 minutes of netball

- 70 minutes on a step machine

- 60 minutes of racquet sports such as squash or tennis (fewer if you play competitively and go hard)

- 60 minutes of aerobics

- 60 minutes of rowing

- 60 minutes of vigorous weight training

- 50 minutes of climbing stairs

- 45 minutes of fast lap swimming

- 30–45 minutes of cycling (the harder you go the less time it takes you)

- 35 minutes of running (at 5 kilometres/hour—if you run slower you must run for longer to burn the same energy)

I'm guessing that, like me, you are short on time so fitting in daily exercise to burn that amount of energy is tough. But you'll see that the harder you work the less time you need to spend. For most of us, this is the key to success in our exercise regimen—work harder in less time. This is also why we should separate activity and exercise—build lots of slow-burn activity into every day, and then add the energy-burn boost of a few intense exercise sessions. Understanding the FITT principles will help you to do just that.

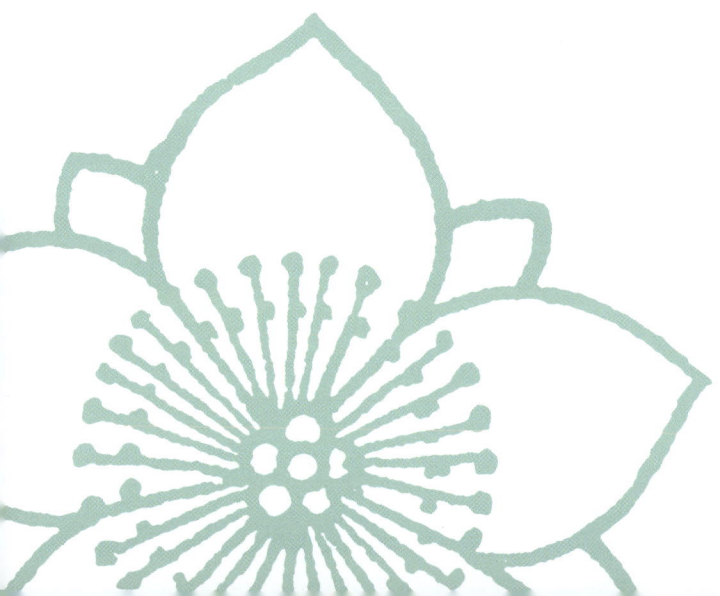

FITT Principles

F requency = the number of times in the week that you exercise
I ntensity = how hard you work during the exercise
T ime = how long you exercise for
T ype = what sort of exercise you do

These are the four basic variables of exercise that come together to represent how many kilojoules you burn, how much fat you burn and ultimately how fit you become. Plan for these four things for an effective exercise program.

Total energy burned = frequency x intensity x time

There's no reason to have a complicated training plan, unless you're training for a specific event or are a professional sportsperson. The formula puts it in perspective. If you increase one of the three factors you'll increase your energy output. Increase more than one factor and you're well on your way to a strong fit body.

So, the more times in the week you work out (frequency) the more kilojoules you will burn that week. The harder you go during the workout (intensity) the more kilojoules you will burn in that workout. The longer you exercise for, the more kilojoules you will burn during that workout. And the more kilojoules you burn the better for weight control, both fat loss and prevention of fat gain.

This formula also tells you that if you cannot increase one of these factors then increase one of the others to get results. For example, if you are struggling to find workout space in your diary, go for high-intensity exercise. A 20-minute early morning run, a 45-minute indoor cycling class at your local gym, or a fast-paced game of squash two or three times a week are all great options for you. For those of you who cannot or hate to do high-intensity exercise, you must find additional time or manage more exercise sessions through your week. So, you get the idea—if one factor goes down raise the bar on at least one other variable.

Key FITT concepts

- The less time you have, the harder you need to work

- If you do gentler, less intense forms of exercise you need to do them more often and for longer each time

- Every session of exercise is valuable, regardless of how long, how hard or how frequent

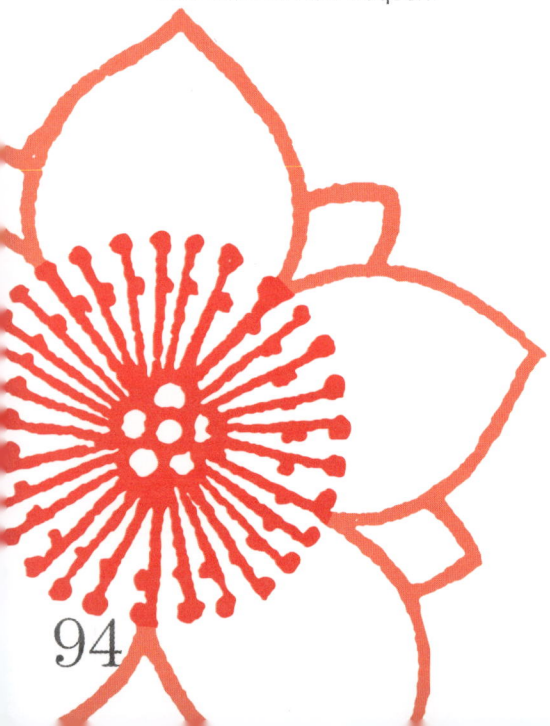

Exercise — which ones?

What will I enjoy doing? Forcing yourself to go running will never last if you truly hate it. That said, you won't always love your chosen exercise— there will be times when you have to motivate yourself to do it. But more often than not, once into your workout you'll enjoy it and will feel fantastic afterwards.

Do I have any physical limitations? Do you have a bad knee that excludes running, or are you pregnant which rules out high impact activities? Obviously, painful arthritis limits what movements you can do. Ask a health or fitness professional to help you choose the best exercise for your condition.

What facilities do I need? We can put on running shoes and head out the door for a walk or run, but many other exercise types require a gym, dance club, sports club or swimming pool. If you have to travel too far, the chances of you keeping up a long-term commitment are greatly reduced.

What will it cost and can I afford it? Don't allow cost to be prohibitive to your new healthier active life. Be very sure that if you sign up for an expensive luxury gym you'll continue to be happy paying that fee a year from now. There are many health clubs and gyms today that are comfortably affordable and have all the facilities you need without the bells and whistles of the more expensive ones. Of course, working out in the park or on the beach costs you nothing except the price of a decent pair of workout shoes.

You needn't just pick one form of exercise either—in fact, the more the better. That's the whole basis of cross-training. You challenge your body in different ways, work different muscle groups and reduce your chance of overuse injuries that can occur with too much of one form of exercise.

> Every session of exercise is valuable, regardless of how long, how hard or how frequent.

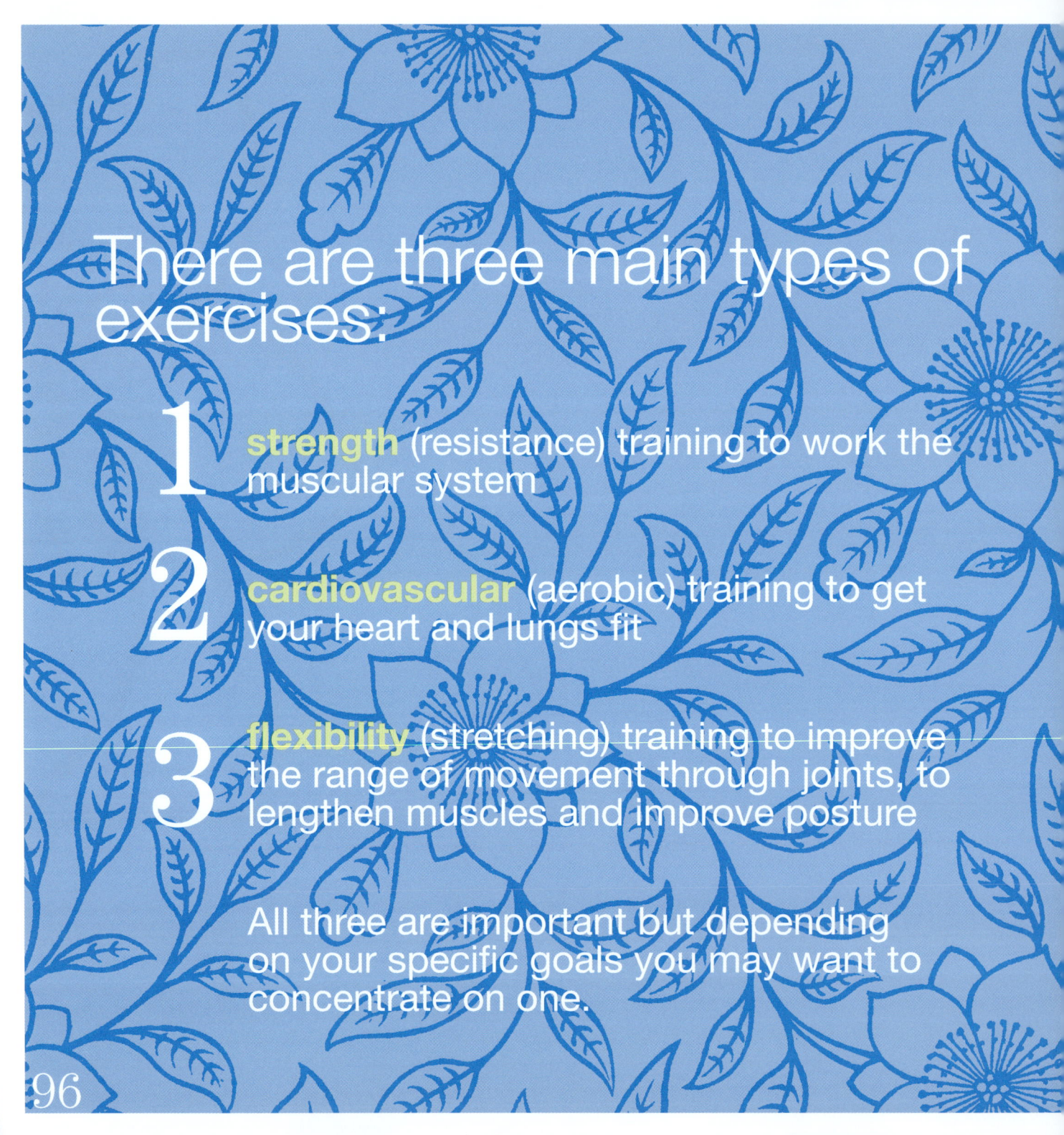

There are three main types of exercises:

1 **strength** (resistance) training to work the muscular system

2 **cardiovascular** (aerobic) training to get your heart and lungs fit

3 **flexibility** (stretching) training to improve the range of movement through joints, to lengthen muscles and improve posture

All three are important but depending on your specific goals you may want to concentrate on one.

Stay strong with strength training

Look in the weights section of any gym and you might expect to find only young men with bulging biceps. Thankfully, that stereotypical image is becoming a thing of the past. It's not that the boys have gone, but there are more women discovering that strength training is often what's missing from their exercise routine. It's arguably the best means we have of really changing the shape of our bodies and it keeps us looking younger by maintaining a strong posture and frame.

Every woman, particularly over the age of 35, should do some form of resistance training on a regular basis. It has nothing to do with developing big muscles—I'm not talking about that level of training or commitment. But if you consider that during the course of our adult life we lose about 50 per cent of our muscle mass, it sheds light on the cause of several age-related problems we commonly face.

"The muscle wastage process is already underway!"

First and foremost, muscles are there to move limbs. Without sufficient strength we would be unable to perform everyday activities. This is what so often happens in our twilight years—reduced muscle size and strength make relatively simple movements a challenge, such as lifting your own body weight out of a chair or opening a can of soup. For many of us this might seem a long way off, but if you are not currently strength training, the muscle wastage process is already underway. For those who think it might be too late, the great news is the research has shown that even seniors can regain some of their previous strength with correct training. It's never too late to start.

But it's not just a matter of how strong you are. Muscle also has a role to play in weight control. If you are struggling with 'middle-age spread', strength training might be your answer. While it's true that our metabolism slows as we age, this can be almost entirely accounted for by the loss in muscle mass. Muscle is active tissue—it burns substantially more energy than fat every minute of the day and night. In other words, if two women have the same weight but different body fat percentage, the one with more muscle and less fat burns more energy every day than her fatter colleague. Over time this makes the woman with more muscle the more likely to remain lean.

If you have been on the dieting merry-go-round for years, losing and regaining weight, this situation is likely to be more pronounced. Losing weight quickly inevitably leads to both muscle and fat loss, but the weight you regain is almost entirely fat. Strength training might just be the solution you need for long-term successful weight control.

" If you are struggling with training just might be your

Our declining muscle mass might also be part of the reason that levels of type-2 diabetes, and its precursor condition insulin resistance, continue to rise in most industrialised countries around the world, including Australia. As well as moving our limbs, muscle plays a very active role in metabolism, particularly of glucose. Muscle takes up glucose from the blood and is the major store of glucose (as glycogen). The more muscle you have, and the more exercised those muscles are, the more efficient this process. This means that fit, strong people are far less likely to develop insulin resistance and type-2 diabetes. This also reduces the risk of added health complications including heart disease.

HOW TO DO IT

Lifting weights is undoubtedly one of the best ways to do strength training, so it is well worth considering joining a gym where a qualified instructor can design an individualised program for you. Working with a personal trainer (if you can afford it) can bring you fantastic results. Bear in mind you needn't do every session with your trainer and they design a program specially for you so it can be money well spent. Many trainers also offer small group training that helps to reduce the cost and some find more fun. Most gyms and leisure centres also run strength training group fitness classes, such as Bodypump®. These can be an excellent and fun way to strength train if you like the group atmosphere. Test out a few different instructors to find one that motivates you and ensures your good technique. Try to attend a technique class first if you are a novice or you may end up feeling lost in the class. Some one-on-one training is far safer to ensure your safety and get you results.

middle-age spread, strength answer. **99**

Those of you that hate the idea of a gym don't need to step inside one in order to strength train. Strength training can be done using hand weights, resistance bags, your body weight or makeshift weights such as bags of rice. Classic exercises such as squats, lunges, push-ups and tricep dips have stood the test of time for good reason—they are effective ways to strength train the major muscle groups using your own body weight as resistance. You can do these at home, in the park or at the beach, during or after the cardio part of your workout. In fact, the exercises I like best are those that simulate our more active ancestral past. This sort of strength training, plus anything that involves lifting, carrying and/or pushing, fits the bill.

Heart to heart with cardio

Cardiovascular exercise is any exercise that makes you a little (or a lot) out of breath. This type of exercise is all about working out the heart, lungs and circulatory system. You should feel your heartbeat quickening and your lungs taking in more air to send the required oxygen to the hardworking muscles. The muscles involved in moving you are of course also getting a workout and this sort of exercise involves a great deal of energy. So, you're burning off kilojoules, many of which will be coming from body fat stores, which is all good news for weight control and improving the shape of your body.

But don't think too much about how much fat you burn during the exercise. It's not that important in the big picture, mainly because for several hours after exercise (particularly intense exercise) your level of fat burning is increased. Given the right food (principally carbs and protein) your body will work to restock the crucial, limited carb stores used up during the exercise— and while it does so a shift towards using up stored fat occurs. So, the benefits of your workout continue long after the hard work is over.

What is important is to keep up an intensity that you can cope with for the correct duration. There is no point in going so hard that you collapse in a heap after 5 minutes! To help you manage the intensity of your cardiovascular workouts there is no need for fancy or expensive equipment. The rate of perceived exertion (RPE) scale is ideal and is used by fitness instructors the world over to guide people in their workouts.

The wonderful thing about RPE is that it works for athletes and complete beginners—it's all down to how you feel. This means that an RPE of 8 may be fast running to some, but to novice exercisers this may be brisk walking. The examples given here are only to give you the idea.

For most of your cardio workouts aim to work at around levels 5 and 6. Once you are more experienced you can then try to complete short intervals at higher intensities. This is the basis of interval training. For example, you could walk for 3 minutes at around level 5, then for the following 1 minute you increase to a run and feel your exertion move up to around level 8. You then follow this with a recovery back to level 5 for another round. This pushes your fitness and increases the energy burn without having to work at uncomfortably high levels for too long.

The latest research even shows that interval training increases the amount of fat you can burn during the course of the workout. An Australian study by the University of New South Wales compared two groups of women: one group exercised at a steady pace for 40 minutes, while the other followed a cycle of 8 seconds sprinting with 12 seconds at a slower gentler level for a total of 20 minutes. The women in the interval training group lost three times as much fat as the other women, despite spending less time overall on the exercise! More fat in less time. The other amazing result from this research was that rather than lose fat from all over as tends to happen when we exercise, the interval training women lost more fat from their legs and bums. Previously it was thought that 'spot reducing' fat from specific areas was impossible. The researchers involved explained the result as being an effect unique to this sprinting style of exercise. A short bout of such high-intensity exercise releases chemical compounds into your body called catecholamines—these stimulate fat from under the skin and in the muscles to be used to fuel the exercise. Apply the interval-training concept to running, cycling, rowing or swimming—it's a very effective way of working out.

HOW TO DO IT

Brisk walking, jogging, running, indoor and outdoor cycling, rowing, swimming, aerobics, gym cardio machines, most team sports, racquet sports, skiing and all forms of dancing are great examples of cardio exercise. Many of these also incorporate strength training at the same time, but the primary focus is cardio fitness. Find what you like, what is available to you, what you can afford to do—and then do it regularly!

Please forget about working out in your 'fat-burning zone'! It's usually quoted at around 60 per cent of your maximal heart rate. This idea came about because the ratio of fat to carbohydrate you burn during exercise changes with the intensity. As the intensity increases you burn a larger percentage of carbohydrate because this provides more immediate energy. Fat is the long, slow burner and takes time to release its energy. The theory was that we should keep the intensity of a workout down in order to increase the ratio of fat being burned. But the truth is that the more intense the workout, the more kilojoules are burned overall. The ratio of fat might have gone down, but more total fat, more carbohydrate and more overall energy have been burned.

Rate of Perceived Exertion (RPE) scale

LEVEL	EXERTION	HOW I FEEL
1	None	Relaxed and sitting comfortably
2	Minimal	Could do this all day
3	Moderate	Getting warmer
4	Noticeable	Starting to sweat and can feel my heart rate increasing but feeling good—could do this for a while
5	Considerable	Sweating, breathing harder but still able to talk

LEVEL	EXERTION	HOW I FEEL
6	Strong	Can still talk but am getting a little breathless
7	Stronger	Breathing and sweating hard—this is tough
8	Very strong	Can no longer hold a conversation. Can only keep this up for a very short time
9	Very, very strong	Legs feel heavy, gasping for air and can only last a few seconds
10	Maximal	Absolutely awful! I have to slow down

Staying strong and flexible

Flexibility is often overlooked in an exercise regime, probably because it doesn't help with weight loss. But maintaining flexibility, particularly as we age, is key to maintaining good mobility, posture, preventing and treating back problems and reducing the risk of injury from the other forms of exercise we do. Just as you feel fantastic after a good massage or manipulation from your chiropractor or physio, your body feels wonderful after a really good stretch class.

Whether or not you need to stretch after your warm-up is still debated and the conclusion seems to be that if it feels good then do it. But at the end of the workout it's a must. Muscles contract and shorten during a workout so a proper cool down to re-lengthen them will help alleviate soreness one or two days later and reduce the chance of injury. If you don't stretch regularly, you risk permanent shortening of some muscle groups, decreased range of movement in joints, and ultimately aches and pains from incorrect posture and alignment.

Stretch regularly and the benefits include:

- **Improved flexibility** This in turn makes every movement of your body more comfortable.

- **Increased range of movement through your joints** Especially as you get older this can help to keep you mobile and maintain good balance.

- **Stress management** Being stressed can make your muscles tense and contract. Nothing beats a good stretch to unwind and de-stress.

- **Better posture** Too much time in a chair, especially on the computer, often causes short, tight hip flexors and chest muscles. This can pull your skeleton out of alignment. Stretching and improved flexibility help you to look taller, slimmer and be free of back pain.

- **Improved circulation** Stretching increases the blood flow through the muscles. This can help recovery after a workout by delivering oxygen and nutrients more quickly and clearing out waste by-products such as lactic acid, responsible for muscle soreness.

- **Fewer injuries** A lithe body can better cope with the demands of everyday life including exercise.

How to do it

Classes such as yoga, Pilates and BodyBalance™ incorporate aspects of both strength and flexibility training, or you can attend a pure stretch class— the best ones tend to be at good dance schools. Find the time to attend once a week and you'll find not only your body will benefit, but also your mind. Stretching is one the best ways to de-stress and get rid of the week's built-up tension.

'**I found that when I discovered Pilates through injury, my body changed significantly in shape and strength within a short period of time ... I had been told to stop all high-impact activity due to knee surgery. It really made a huge difference to my health, both physically and mentally.**' Joan, 30s, British

Five stretches for everyday

Here's an easy sequence of five stretches to build into your day without really having to try. They are especially good for those of us who spend much of the day deskbound. You could do these while you're waiting for the kettle to boil or for your document to print. Hold each stretch for at least 15 seconds, preferably 30.

1 Spinal twist

Sit up tall in your chair on your seat bones, lift your breastbone and lengthen your spine. Turn to look over one shoulder, pulling on the armrest with your opposite hand to increase the stretch. Repeat on the other side.

2 Chest and shoulder opener

Sit or stand 'tall' and join your hands behind your back. With your palms together straighten your arms and lift your hands away from you, feeling the stretch across the front of the shoulders and chest.

3 Forward hang

Stand up and with feet shoulder-distance apart, reach up high to the ceiling with both hands. Exhale and 'forward fold' as if trying to touch your toes. Allow your body to hang, lifting your tailbone, and allow the upper body to relax into the stretch. Breathe. This is great for releasing the lower back and lengthening the hamstrings.

4 Hip opener

Step one foot back as far as you can, taking your hands onto the floor either side of your front foot. Straighten your back leg so it is almost parallel to the floor and ensure your front knee stays directly over your ankle and doesn't sneak forward. Feel the stretch through the extended hip.

5 Downward dog

A favourite yoga move, this does wonders for the backs of the legs right down to your heels. From the hip opener stretch, step the other foot back so that your feet are about hip distance apart and then try to get your heels onto the floor with both legs straight. Think of lifting your hips and pressing down through your shoulder blades. Repeat the hip opener on the other leg and then repeat the downward dog once more. Finish by stepping one foot back between your hands, then the other foot, and rolling up to standing. Take a big breath in and out, circling your arms over your head and back as you do so, centre yourself with beautiful posture and you're done.

Choosing the right exercise

YOUR SITUATION	BEST EXERCISE CHOICES
I want to lose weight	Focus on cardio exercise, such as brisk walking, jogging, cycling, rowing, dance and most sports fit the bill. Incorporate interval training to increase fat burn in less time.
I want to tone up and improve my shape	Strength training, such as weights or resistance exercises. Pilates and more active yoga classes.
I want stress relief and relaxation	Mind–body style classes, for example BodyBalance™ or yoga.
I need to relieve built-up tension and frustration	Cardio cardio cardio! You can't beat it for getting rid of anger, tension and frustration. Boxing, martial arts and boot camp classes are also fantastic.
I want to improve my posture and pelvic floor strength	Pilates, BodyBalance™, training on Bosu (like half a ball—flat on one side and domed on the other) or fitball, Alexander technique.
I want to meet people and socialise while I exercise	Team sports, sports clubs, for example tennis and squash clubs, group exercise classes, dance classes.

YOUR SITUATION

I travel a lot and need to fit exercise into my busy schedule

I am very overweight and find it uncomfortable to exercise

I have a bad back/knees/other joint problems

I am very thin and would like to gain weight but as muscle not fat to improve my shape

I hate the idea of exercising for exercise's sake but want to get fit

BEST EXERCISE CHOICES

Running, jogging, brisk walking. All you need do is take a pair of running shoes with you.

Swimming is perfect—it takes pressure off joints but the water adds resistance, providing some strength training at the same time. Also try aqua aerobic classes.

See a physio for a proper assessment of the problem before you undertake any exercise and follow their advice. Pilates taught one-on-one or in a small group can often help those with more serious problems. More often than not exercise helps, so don't be resigned to the sofa.

Strength training is without doubt your answer. Join a gym and work with a personal trainer or attend a weights class. Thin women are also at increased risk of having weak bones— strength training builds and maintains stronger bones.

Try exercise incorporated into a game. Team sports or competitive sports, such as tennis or squash. Or try something different such as a dance class where skill and technique can be your focus. Plus they are lots of fun.

Finding the motivation to move

'I think about going to the gym tomorrow!' Abi, 30s, British

Is this you?

- You look forward to exercising.
- You feel grumpy and resentful if you have to forego a workout.
- You'll get up extra early if that's the only way to fit in a session, even in winter or on a public holiday.
- You prefer going to the gym than having drinks with colleagues after work.
- You think walking for an hour is a nice rest.

Not you? Don't despair, you're not alone! Most of us struggle sometimes to find the motivation to get moving and keep moving.

"Make exercise a habit."

INHIBIT THE HABIT

So how can we do it? Undeniably part of the problem is habit. That little word plays such an important part in our lives and rules much of what we do. We are indeed 'creatures of habit'. If you always head to the local bar with your work colleagues at the end of the day for a wind-down glass of chardonnay, that is exactly what you will always feel like doing come that time of day. If you always head straight to the gym for the 6.30 class on a Tuesday night, that too becomes a habit, and over time it's far easier to keep up than when you first started. So trick number one is: make exercise a habit.

Habits are not formed overnight, so accept that it will take some time. It probably takes even longer to successfully break a habit. Don't treat the inevitable slips back into your old ways as failures—they are all part and parcel of breaking the old habits and creating new ones. As the weeks go by you will find that keeping up your exercise routine becomes easier as you reawaken that active person inside.

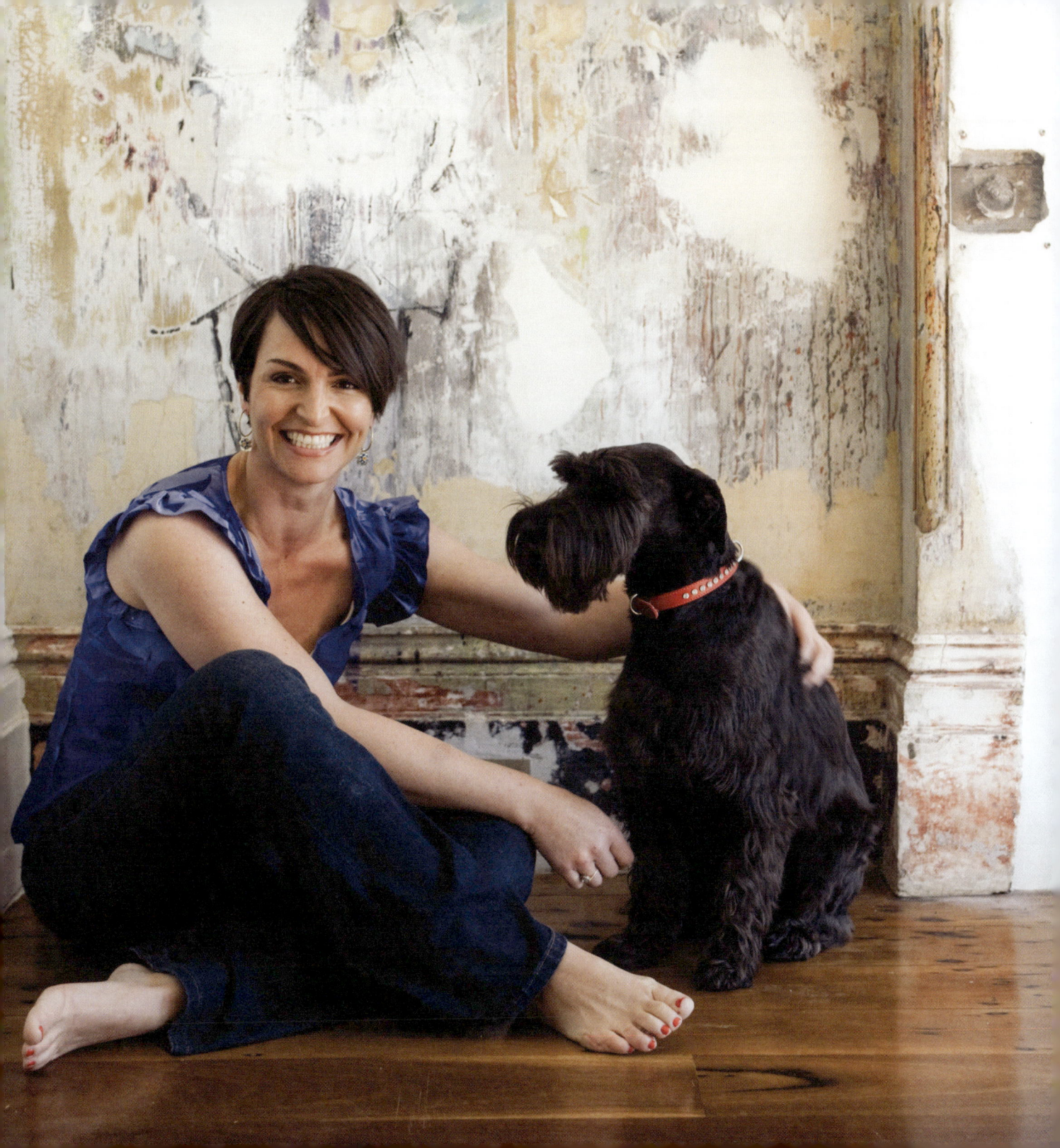

How to break the habit and take control

INSTEAD OF...

Driving to the shop that's 5 mins down the road when you run out of milk

... DO THIS

Walk. It may take 10 minutes longer, but are you really so short on time for this to matter? Not only will you reap the physical benefit, but you'll also be doing your bit for the environment.

INSTEAD OF...

Parking as close as possible to your destination, even if it means driving around 5 minutes longer to secure the spot

... DO THIS

Park a little further away and walk the remainder. Even if it's only across the car park it will instil an active mentality in both you and your family.

INSTEAD OF...

Emailing a colleague in the same building so you don't have to move from your desk

... DO THIS

Get up and take a walk down the hall! It's even better if you have to venture up a flight of stairs or two. Your personal communication will be more effective and you'll burn a few kilojoules along the way—a win-win situation!

INSTEAD OF...

Staying up late at night watching TV only to feel exhausted the next morning. Staying in bed until the last minute before you have to start a day's work

... DO THIS

Skip late night TV and get up earlier to fit in a 30-minute brisk walk before work. You'll instantly feel better and more energised for the rest of the day.

INSTEAD OF...

Standing still on escalators and travelators (balancing a stroller, being injured or elderly or carrying a heavy load I'll except as valid excuses)

... DO THIS

Walk or use the stairs whenever possible. When you're on the moving device at least keep moving yourself!

INSTEAD OF...

Spending hours at your desk without getting up to move

Vegging in front of the TV every night in an exhausted mental state

Always looking for a seat on the bus, the train, or in a waiting room

... DO THIS

Every hour or so get up and walk around the office, have a stretch or at least stand while making phone calls. Try to take a walk round the block at lunchtime or even better head to the gym for a mid-day workout or to the pool for a swim. You might even find your work productivity goes up as your brain and body are energised.

Recognise the difference between mental and physical exhaustion. You may be mentally exhausted from work or a stressful day with the kids, but this is not physical exhaustion. Fit in a half-hour walk, head for a workout or put on a fitness DVD before you settle down in front of the TV. Do some activity while watching TV, for example the ironing or a stretch or resistance training routine.

Don't sit when you can stand and don't stand when you can walk. Standing involves muscular activity to hold you upright and to balance. When you walk the energy level jumps again. Always choose the most active level possible.

113

The key to achieving fitness is to become the sort of person who always chooses the active option, who chooses to be an active participant in life. You are the one who offers to walk to the shop for takeaway coffees. You are the one to pop down the stairs to deliver something to a colleague. You are the one who leaps at the chance to take part in a charity fun run. You are the one who stuffs her high heels in her bag and walks to work in her runners. You are the one who puts on some music and dances round the living room with the giggling three-year-old. Whatever it may be, grab every opportunity to get moving.

"Live
to
move"

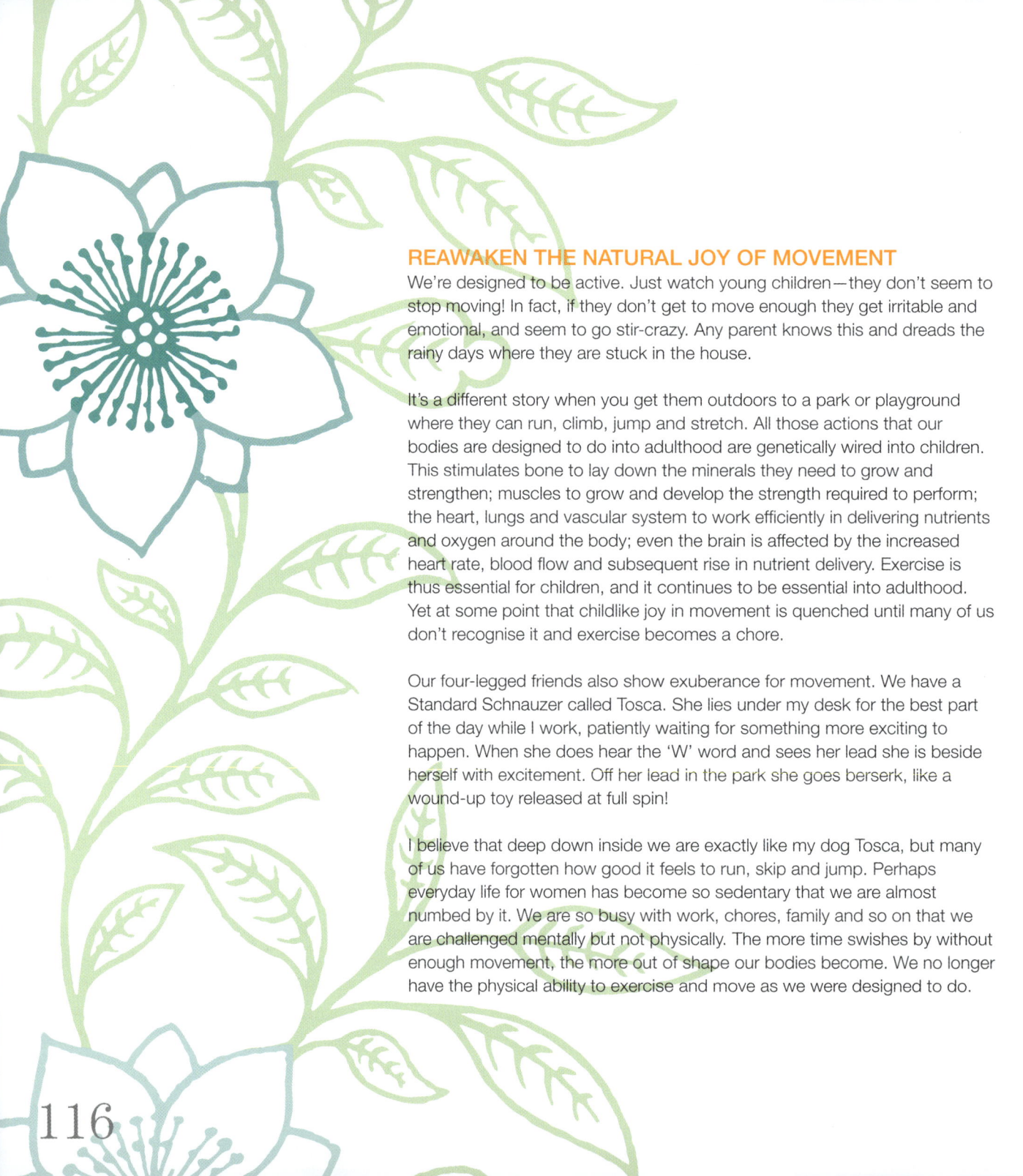

REAWAKEN THE NATURAL JOY OF MOVEMENT

We're designed to be active. Just watch young children—they don't seem to stop moving! In fact, if they don't get to move enough they get irritable and emotional, and seem to go stir-crazy. Any parent knows this and dreads the rainy days where they are stuck in the house.

It's a different story when you get them outdoors to a park or playground where they can run, climb, jump and stretch. All those actions that our bodies are designed to do into adulthood are genetically wired into children. This stimulates bone to lay down the minerals they need to grow and strengthen; muscles to grow and develop the strength required to perform; the heart, lungs and vascular system to work efficiently in delivering nutrients and oxygen around the body; even the brain is affected by the increased heart rate, blood flow and subsequent rise in nutrient delivery. Exercise is thus essential for children, and it continues to be essential into adulthood. Yet at some point that childlike joy in movement is quenched until many of us don't recognise it and exercise becomes a chore.

Our four-legged friends also show exuberance for movement. We have a Standard Schnauzer called Tosca. She lies under my desk for the best part of the day while I work, patiently waiting for something more exciting to happen. When she does hear the 'W' word and sees her lead she is beside herself with excitement. Off her lead in the park she goes berserk, like a wound-up toy released at full spin!

I believe that deep down inside we are exactly like my dog Tosca, but many of us have forgotten how good it feels to run, skip and jump. Perhaps everyday life for women has become so sedentary that we are almost numbed by it. We are so busy with work, chores, family and so on that we are challenged mentally but not physically. The more time swishes by without enough movement, the more out of shape our bodies become. We no longer have the physical ability to exercise and move as we were designed to do.

"Grab every opportunity to get moving. "

We lose muscle, joint flexibility and our heart and lungs cannot support the increased work demands that the activity brings. Exercise becomes difficult and uncomfortable. If you are very overweight you have the added difficulty of stress placed on your joints, muscular system and heart.

Those of you who exercise regularly know how good you feel after a workout. Equally, you know how bad you feel when you don't find the time for workouts. Together these factors provide serious motivation for you to keep it up. But for the out-of-shape woman who hasn't exercised in years it's a different set of circumstances. If this is you, you might feel dreadful after exercising, particularly if you pushed yourself too hard. Your body is physically unable to cope and the shock to the system may leave you exhausted and even physically sick. A day or two later you feel like you've been hit by a bus. Every muscle in your body aches and it's an effort to even get out of bed. It's little wonder that so many newcomers to exercise give up pretty quickly.

But you can turn it around! If you reawaken your natural joy in movement you are more than halfway to becoming the active woman you desire to be. Start slowly and you will get over the initial discomfort. Think about being more active from day to day and then add formal exercise sessions. From there, build how much you do, how hard you work and before long being active will simply be a part of who you are and not something you have to try to be.

Move with the groove

Music and rhythm are at the very heart of us. Native peoples around the world sing, dance and make music of some kind. It's often integral to their cultural identity. Just picture the Masai warriors of Kenya playing their bongo-style drums while dancing and singing around the fire. Is this all that different to feeling the urge to dance to a favourite song? We may not all like the same music, and some of us are far more musical than others, but almost everyone is moved in some way by music and in turn music encourages us to move. Group exercise uses music to motivate and encourage you during a class. It may not be what you'd play at home, but a good class will have music that pushes you to work harder, or relax in the moment, or simply get you moving. I have a program of 'power songs' on my MP3 player for when I go running. When I'm flagging during my run I can hit the button and my power songs kick in. It really works.

Bring your buddies

Some people prefer to work out alone and the idea of a group program appals them. If this is you then solo walking, running, cycling, kayaking or swimming will work well. Others work harder and more consistently when exercising with a group or another person. You can join a fitness class—the energy in the room of a good class is infectious. Or you can simply team up with your partner or a friend to go walking or running. Of course, any sort of team sport is fantastic for those who are both competitive and like to exercise with others.

We are social creatures for the most part and if you can make exercise and activity a part of your social life you'll find it much easier to keep it up. Weekend or after-work tennis, squash, beach volleyball, netball, group mountain-bike riding or road cycling, running clubs or ballroom/salsa and any other style of dancing are all great social sports/exercise. You may also consider hiring a personal trainer. A good one will have excellent motivational skills and will use several of these other techniques to push you to give your best. Many trainers now run sessions for pairs or small groups of like-minded people. Some people find this more enjoyable and it can reduce the costs.

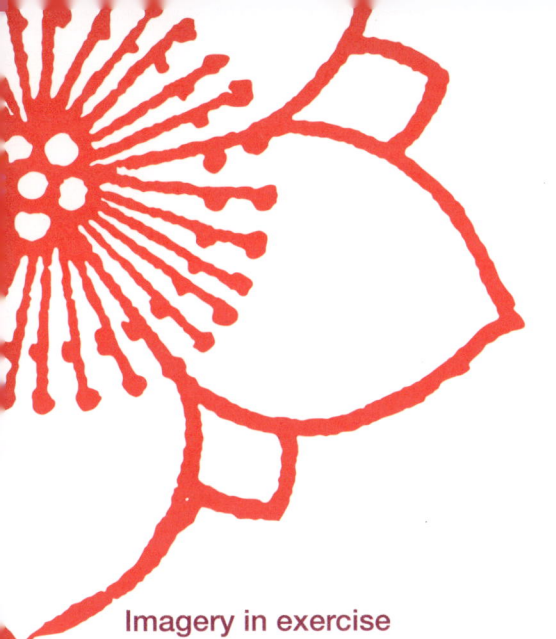
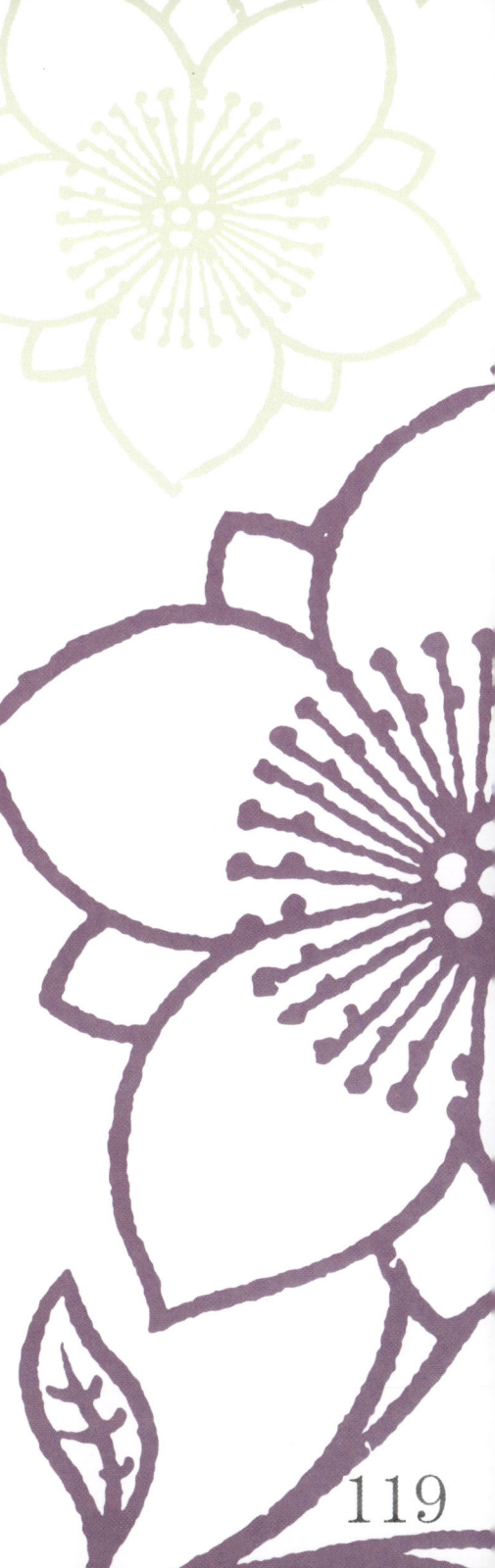

Imagery in exercise

Mental imagery can be a powerful motivational technique to help you exercise harder and keep going during a workout. If you are struggling to head out the door for your workout, try visualising all the good things that happen inside your body when you exercise. Imagine the way that you'll feel when exercising well and how energised and fantastic you'll feel once the workout is over. Imagine your body burning fat, your heart pumping stronger, the blood coursing through your veins and delivering oxygen and nutrients to your working muscles. This not only helps you to work harder but also drives out the other thoughts of the day that may be dominating your mind. It's a fantastic way to help relieve stress and clear your mind.

Know your mantra

A school friend of mine was a meditation enthusiast. When I asked her how she gets into her meditative state, she said she chants her own mantra inside her head. I won't profess to know much about meditation, so forgive my simple explanation but clearly the mantra helps her to achieve a different level of consciousness, awareness or whatever you wish to call it. Sportspeople and athletes often use a similar technique—Lleyton Hewitt's shout of 'Come on!' is essentially his motivating mantra. Nike's very successful advertising campaign has the brilliant *Just do it!* and this works beautifully as a mantra to get yourself up and moving. On the facing wall of the exercise studio in my gym they have another Nike slogan: *I can*. I will. I am. Steal one of these (or all of them!) or make up your own. Use your mantra during your workout, particularly when it's getting tough and you need to push to get to the next level. It really does work.

119

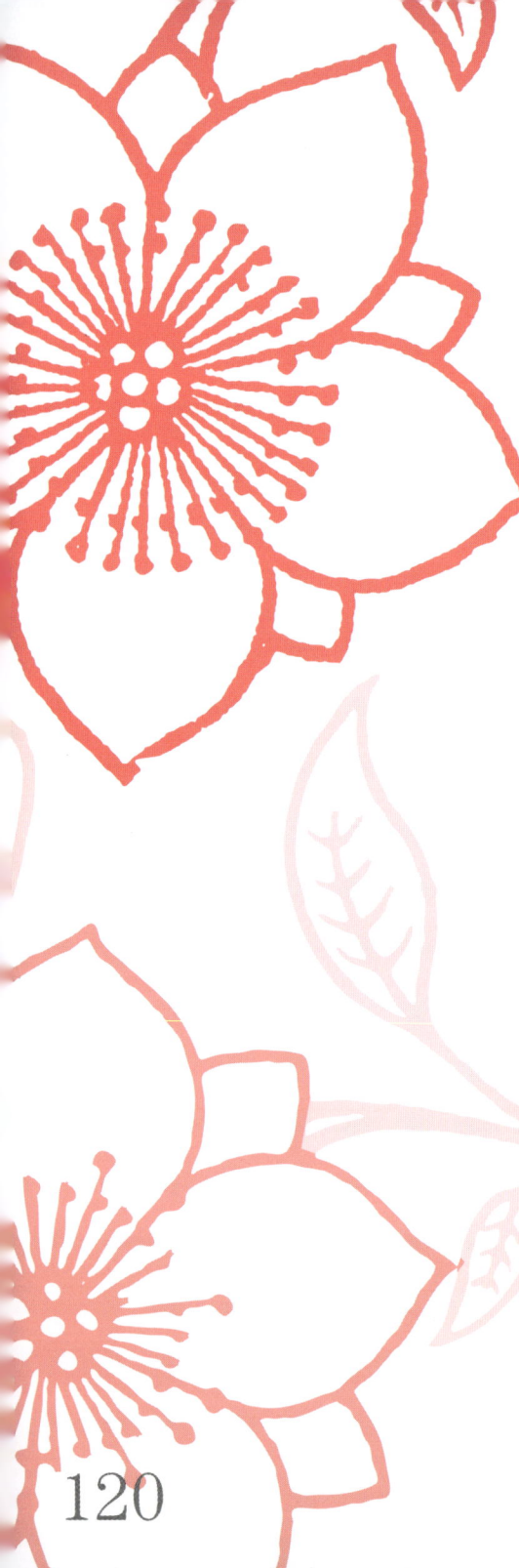

Don't let exercise run you down

There's no doubt most of us need to move more, but there are also dangers from exercising too much. Overtraining affects you both mentally and physically. You hit a point where more exercise actually depresses your immune system instead of strengthening it, and your health starts to deteriorate. You're more likely to catch colds and flu, your skin can become dehydrated, and skin conditions such as eczema and psoriasis can flare up. You are likely to feel lethargic even on waking, and you may find that your weight even increases due to your body craving more and more food. Mentally, you may find yourself obsessing over whether or not you have completed enough exercise. You find that your workouts get priority over everything else. I realised an old friend of mine was becoming too exercise-obsessed after she told me she couldn't pick up her fiancé from the airport after he'd been away with work for three weeks because she had to fit in her daily run. It is admirable and desirable to place a good level of importance on your exercise, but don't allow it take over your life. Exercise should enhance your life, not run it. It's about getting the balance right.

'I was once pretty obsessed with exercise as a weight control method. I had an unexpected liberating experience whereby I burnt myself quite badly and was unable to exercise for a couple of months. A number of positive things came out of this. I discovered my body shape didn't change too much (I thought I would turn into a big baboon) and in fact I developed more feminine softness, which I love. Even more liberating was that I didn't obsess about food so much because my appetite dropped off. I now exercise a lot less so my appetite is not so aggressive, and consequently I have more spare time!'
Kath, 30s, New Zealander

"

Exercise should enhance your life, not run it.

"

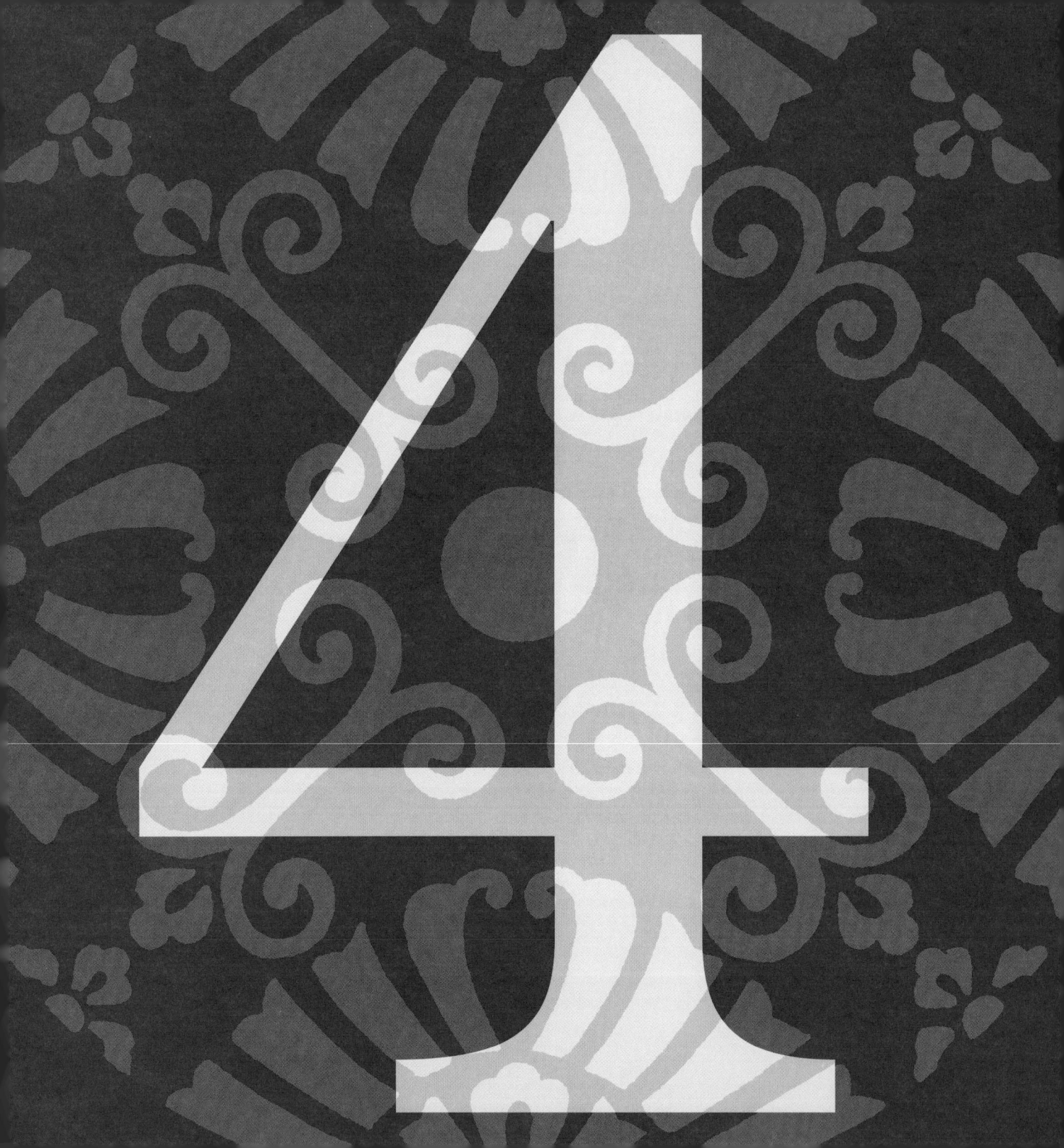

Make it happen

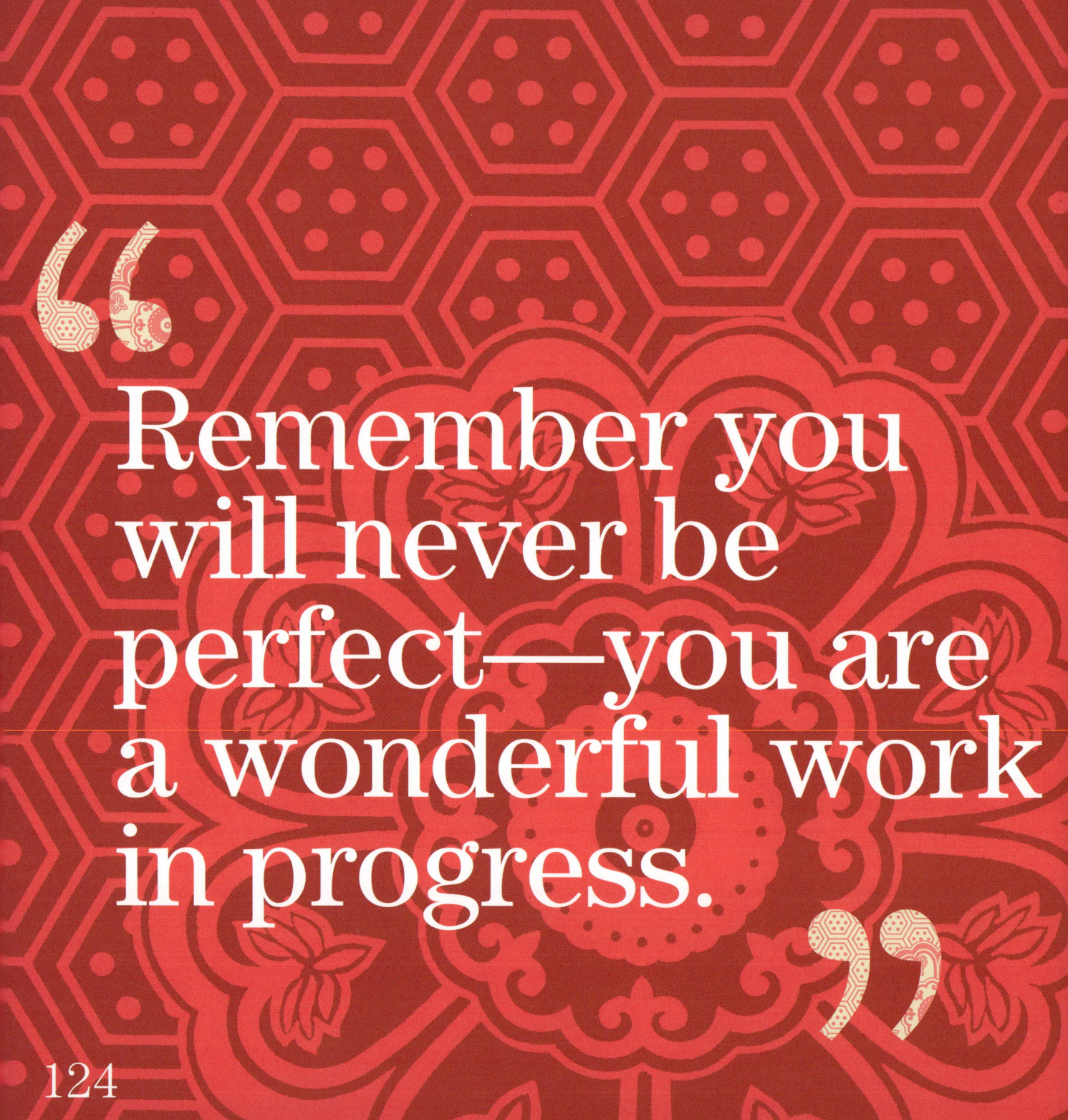

"Remember you will never be perfect—you are a wonderful work in progress."

Most of us attempt to do everything at once, usually on a Monday. 'On Monday I will start my diet, stop eating chocolate, go to the gym every night, give up my nightly glass of wine, never eat lollies in the car again …', and the list goes on. It's no wonder that a week or two down the track it's all too hard and you give up. It's too much too soon. The answer is to prioritise and remember you will never be perfect—you are a wonderful work in progress. There will always be periods in your life when you have to give your lifestyle and diet more attention to get it back on track, and periods when things slip because you haven't been willing or able to give yourself such attention. Accept these cycles. As long as you regularly reassess and get back on track, you will meet your potential for looking and feeling your best.

Checklist of priorities

1 Focus first on the foods that you eat. Look for where improvements can be made. Go back over chapter 1 for help and explore chapter 5 for inspiration.

2 Take a good hard look at how active you are from day to day. Use the goal section in this chapter (p. 128) to help you to build more activity into your life. Check the tips in chapter 3 for loads of ideas on getting more movement into your day.

3 Look at your eating behaviours and consider whether they are holding you back. If emotional eating is a real problem, concentrate on it. Re-read 'Eight great strategies to reduce emotional and binge eating' (p. 78) in chapter 2.

4 Add formal exercise sessions to inject a serious boost to your fitness, strength, toning and energy output. If you're still having trouble deciding what's the best choice for you, go back over the options set out in chapter 3.

5 If you are eating the right foods and doing the right activity and exercise (or as much as you can manage) yet still seem to be having trouble losing weight, try to reduce your portion sizes. Portions are undoubtedly a problem, but I usually don't like to set portion sizes for people as it teaches an external cue to eating rather than an internal one. If you eat the right foods and move in the right way, you should be able to use your own appetite and satiation cues to guide you towards the right amount for you. But I know some women need to control portion size as it can take a long time to learn to 'hear' those internal cues.

You may find that you are already fairly strong in one or more of the areas in this list. That makes it easy—you can focus on the rest. If you have a bit of work to do in all these areas, start with the changes that are likely to have the biggest impact.

Goals should motivate you,

Go for goal

Goal-setting is all about deciding where you want to be and how you are going to get there. If you vaguely say, 'I want to lose weight, get fitter and eat better' then a few months later it's likely nothing will have changed. To get results you have to set yourself goals.

The key to effective goal-setting is to make them SMART.

S pecific
M easurable
A chievable
R elevant
T ime-based

Specific Clearly define what you want to achieve. For example

- 'I want to lose weight' becomes 'I want to lose 2 centimetres from my waist.'
- 'I want to be fitter' becomes 'I want to be able to run continuously for 20 minutes.'

Then decide how you are going to achieve your goal. Prioritise so you're not trying to change too many things at once.

not discourage you.

Measurable A goal can't be reached unless you can measure it. This will also help you to work towards long-term goals as you can measure your progress along the way. For example, if your goal is to run a half marathon, you can measure each incremental training step by setting measurable kilometre running goals. If you have a lot of weight to lose then you should break it down into smaller steps of centimetres lost from your waist or kilos lost on the scale each month. This will help to spur you on to the final goal.

Achievable Set goals you can realistically achieve or you'll set yourself up for failure and disappointment. A body like Elle McPherson is a dream not a goal. Goals should motivate you, not serve to discourage you when you don't get anywhere near them. Set goals that stretch you, certainly, but that are within your reach.

Relevant Try to make all your goals work towards the same result. Create an ultimate aim, if you like, for where you want to get to and then decide which goals are most relevant to get you there. For example, if your aim is to lose 10 kilos and take part in a major fun run next year, then setting a goal to attend a yoga class is not relevant. It's still good for you, but it's not the best exercise to help you achieve your particular aim.

Time-based Most of us need deadlines to make a project happen. It's just the same for our own life projects. If you really want to change the way you eat and move, then set time limits for accomplishing each goal. Start now, this minute, and decide on the time goal. 'I will lose 2 centimetres from my waist' becomes 'I will lose 2 centimetres from my waist by this date next month.'

Commit your goals to paper. Having them in your head is not good enough. It's a good idea to have short-term goals that you can work on this coming week, medium-term ones for the month and long-term goals that will take you several months or up to a year to achieve. Definitive and careful planning is required, so you have to take them seriously.

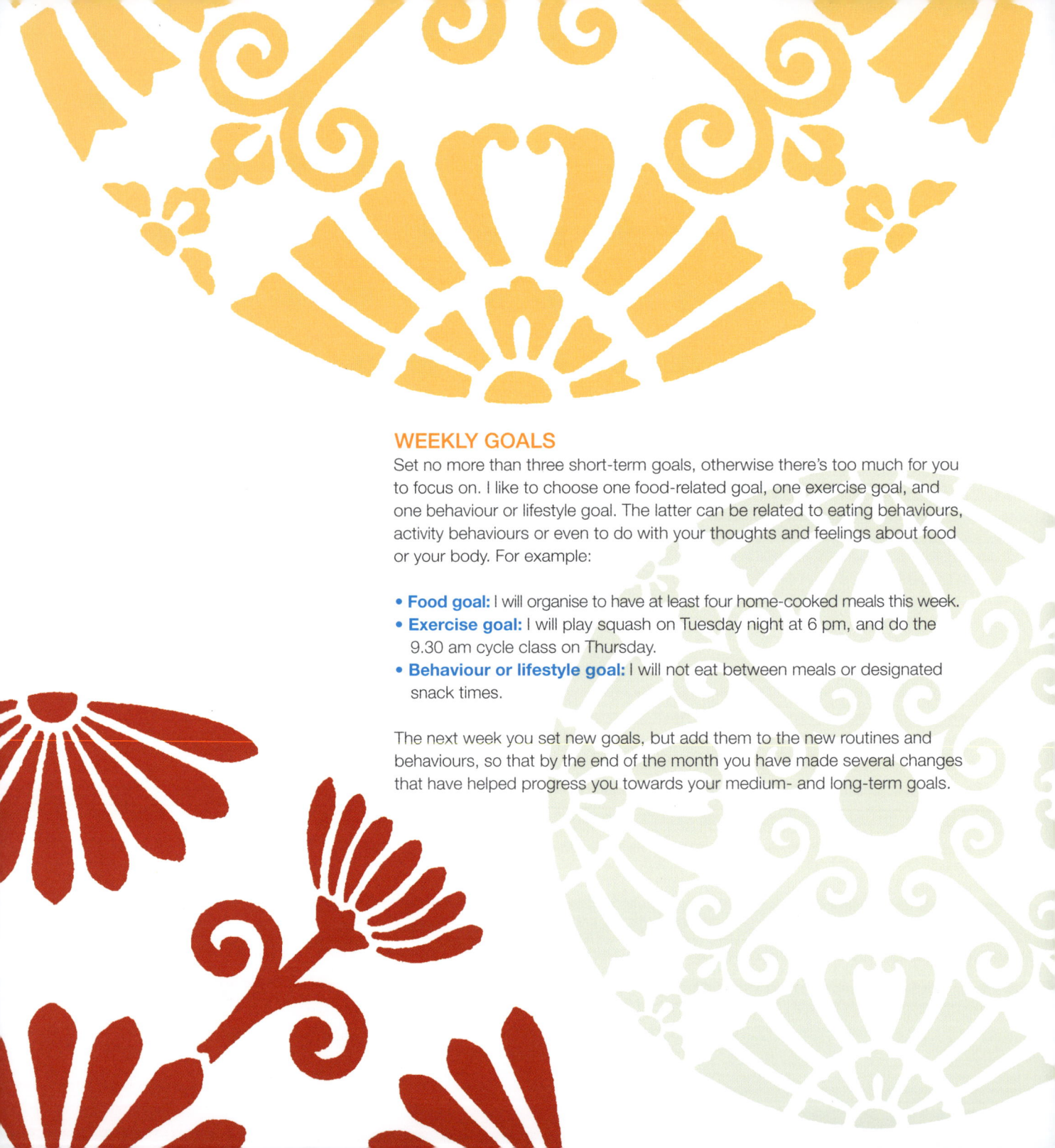

WEEKLY GOALS

Set no more than three short-term goals, otherwise there's too much for you to focus on. I like to choose one food-related goal, one exercise goal, and one behaviour or lifestyle goal. The latter can be related to eating behaviours, activity behaviours or even to do with your thoughts and feelings about food or your body. For example:

- **Food goal:** I will organise to have at least four home-cooked meals this week.
- **Exercise goal:** I will play squash on Tuesday night at 6 pm, and do the 9.30 am cycle class on Thursday.
- **Behaviour or lifestyle goal:** I will not eat between meals or designated snack times.

The next week you set new goals, but add them to the new routines and behaviours, so that by the end of the month you have made several changes that have helped progress you towards your medium- and long-term goals.

MONTHLY GOALS

If your goal is to lose weight or tone up and lose body fat, these goals are best kept for the medium to long term. Weekly changes are often not measurable as our weight naturally fluctuates by a couple of kilos, potentially masking any real change, and body fat percentages and tape measurements really need a longer period of time to show differences.

Fitness goals are also better as monthly targets: running, cycling or swimming a certain distance or time, weight that can be lifted or repetitions you can achieve, or even attendance at a dance class. These goals need not be so specific as the short-term ones, but should be a clear step towards your mission statement. For example: by the end of the month my goal is to lose 2 centimetres from my waist, be able to cycle continuously for 30 minutes and to attend yoga once a week.

YOUR ULTIMATE AIM

This is your long-term goal. It's where you want to be by Christmas, your birthday, a friend's wedding or simply x number of months down the line. Having a specific event can be helpful, as long as when you reach it you don't throw in the towel and return to your old ways! Instead, re-evaluate and set the next set of goals.

Monitoring progress

How you monitor your progress obviously depends on your goal. It's usually best to use more than one means of monitoring. If fitness and toning are what you're after, then measure your strength, your flexibility, your cardio fitness and perhaps do tape measurements. If you want to focus on changing eating habits and your relationship with food, a checklist of behaviours or personal statements true to you would work best. If you're hoping to lose weight, obviously monitoring is important, but it is essential that you don't use weight loss alone, if at all. Let's go through the most common monitoring tools to help you decide which might suit you best.

WEIGHT

Weight is the most common means of assessing progress for most people, whether you want to lose a couple of kilos and tone up, or have a lot of weight to lose. It's fine, provided you understand what weight tells you, and that it continues to be a positive motivation rather than becoming an obsession. I have spoken to many women over the years who have become so obsessed with weight that they have to measure it every morning and their mood for the day is set by the result. Day-to-day fluid shifts and other

"Weighing yourself every you nothing about changes

normal changes affect our weight by as much as 2 kg. Clearly, weighing yourself every morning is crazy and will tell you nothing about changes to your body composition. In fact, since muscle weighs more than fat, women who start a strength-training program sometimes find their weight doesn't change, or even goes up by a small amount, yet they can notch in their belt and feel their clothes getting looser. Think of muscle as compact and heavy compared to fat, which is lighter but takes up more space.

Many personal trainers discourage using weight as a progress guide. I agree entirely for women already in the healthy weight range for their height, or who clearly have a large muscle mass to explain their higher weight. If you fall into this category, weight will really not tell you much and you will certainly need a different way of monitoring your progress. But if your weight is well above your healthy weight range, weighing yourself at appropriate intervals is useful because ultimately you do want your weight to come down. There are advantages to weighing: it's easy to do yourself, you don't need fancy equipment and it changes relatively quickly, which gives a good motivation boost (providing it moves in the right direction). Weigh yourself once a month, so that you eliminate the day-to-day fluctuations and get a clearer picture of the direction of change.

morning is crazy and will tell to your body composition. ,,

133

Are you the right weight for you?

The medical definitions of overweight and obese use the body mass index (BMI). You can calculate this for yourself by dividing your weight in kilograms by your height in metres squared.

BMI = weight (kg) ÷ height (m)^2
For example: 60 (kg) ÷ 1.66 (m)^2 = 21.7

Compare where you are in the official definitions for BMI:

Healthy weight   18–24.9
Overweight   25–29.9
Obese   30+

Don't be bound by these definitions. Use them to give you an idea of a healthy weight range for you.

The BMI Formula

Low end of your healthy weight range: weight = 18 x your height^2

High end of your healthy weight range: weight = 24.9 x your height^2

Ready reckoner

Height	Suggested healthy weight range
1.50 m (4 ft 11 in)	41–56 kg (90–123 lbs)
1.55 m (5 ft 1 in)	43–60 kg (95–132 lbs)
1.6 m (5 ft 3 in)	46–64 kg (101–141 lbs)
1.65 m (5 ft 5 in)	49–68 kg (108–150 lbs)
1.7 m (5 ft 7 in)	52–72 kg (115–159 lbs)
1.75 m (5 ft 9 in)	55–76 kg (121–168 lbs)
1.8 m (5 ft 11 in)	58–81 kg (128–179 lbs)
1.85 m (6 ft 1 in)	62–85 kg (137–187 lbs)

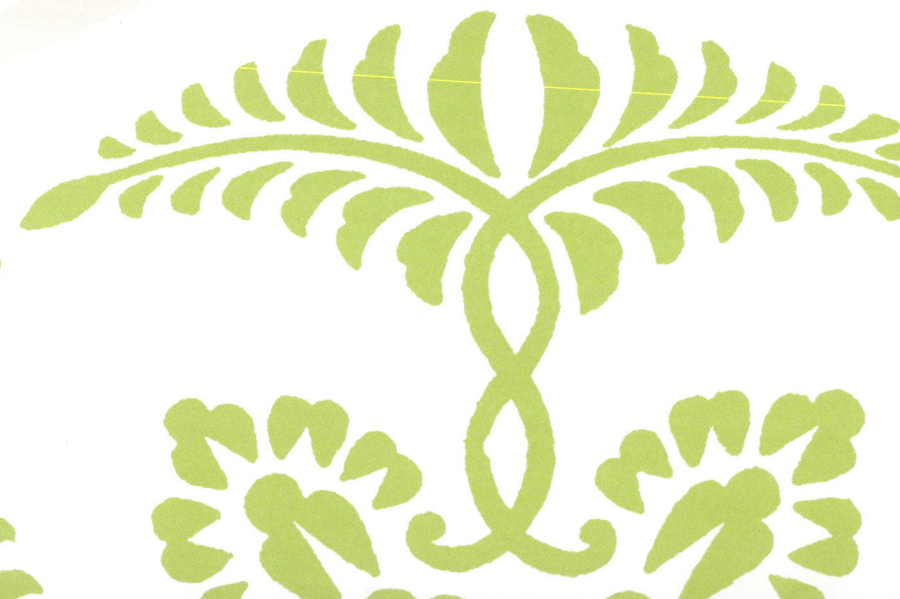

Of course, these official medical definitions don't always reflect how women feel about themselves. I asked women in my survey to choose one of the following words to describe themselves: healthy, fat, skinny, chubby or lean. Of the women who would be officially classified as overweight, a quarter chose the word 'healthy' while the others were divided between 'fat' and 'chubby'. The vast majority of women with BMIs that put them in the official obese category described themselves as fat, but there was still one woman who described herself as healthy. At the other end of the scale most of the women officially categorised as having a healthy weight said they thought they would look better if they lost a couple of kilos. I suspect what these women really mean is that despite being a healthy weight, they would like to be leaner and more toned. For these women weight will not tell them much.

It's important to know that weight does *not* tell the full story. It does not tell us exactly how fat we are, where the fat lies, nor how fit we are. All of these factors matter. Clearly we view ourselves as healthy at different weights. This might be based on your culture (some cultures beautify larger or smaller women), on your family and friend comparisons (being smaller or larger than your family or peers may alter your view of yourself), or simply on how you feel at different weights.

Weight monitoring tips

- There's no such thing as an ideal weight. You have to find what weight is right for you.
- If you need to lose weight, don't set yourself a 'goal weight' but rather a weight range. Weigh yourself no more than once a month and assess your progress alongside a number of other means, such as body fat, waist circumference, fitness goals, clothes size and so on.
- If you do choose to measure your weight, try to view it non-emotionally.
- Be careful to view your body and your weight realistically, neither seeing yourself as fatter than you really are, nor ignoring things if you are overweight or have gained weight.

BODY FAT

There is no doubt that if we could accurately measure it, body fat mass and lean muscle mass would be the best monitoring tool. But we don't have an easy and inexpensive way of measuring it. The best method involves something called a DEXA machine, found mostly in hospitals. It's like a very gentle X-ray of the whole body and is mostly used by doctors to measure bone density for the assessment of osteoporosis. It can also give an accurate measure of both fat and lean mass. These machines are not widely available for body composition measuring, though you may be able to get a referral from your GP or dietitian.

But there are three more accessible ways to analyse body composition:

1 The fit of your clothes. No one gains muscle around their waist so if you are loosening the notches in your belt you can be sure you are gaining body fat! If you live in baggy, loose-fitting, stretchy type clothes it is much easier not to realise what is happening underneath. Buy clothes that fit properly. When things feel tight, do something about it. It's much easier to deal with small changes than to wait until it's a major affair to get back in shape. Likewise, if you are trying to lose weight, the satisfaction of feeling your clothes get looser is great motivation to keep going.

2 Skinfold callipers can be used by a personal trainer, dietitian or health professional specifically trained in body composition measurement to estimate how much fat you have. The accuracy of this method depends on the skill and experience of the trainer, how much fat you have and its distribution, and how many sites on the body are measured. It's not the most pleasant test to have done (who likes to have their fat pinched?), but it will give a reasonably accurate assessment provided it's done correctly.

> # If you live in baggy, loose-fitting, stretchy type clothes it is much easier not to realise what is happening underneath.

3 Body fat monitor scales use a technique called bio-electrical impedance, which measures your body's resistance to the flow of a small electrical current (completely harmless and you won't feel a thing). Resistance to the current is low in lean tissue, where there's lots of water, but high in fat tissue. An estimate of total body water can then be used to calculate your lean body mass. The scale measures your weight at the same time and the amount of fat you have is the difference between your weight and lean body mass. The scales have an inbuilt mathematical formula, based on measurements of hundreds of people, to estimate your body fat level and the results can be amazingly accurate. They are easy to use at home and give a quick reading but since the scales measure your total body water they are affected by how well hydrated you are, the fluid shifts that occur around the body over the course of the day and other factors. They are a good investment, provided you take a few steps to increase their accuracy. Always take a reading at the same time of day, never immediately after exercise or eating a meal, and ensure you are well hydrated.

> **From a health perspective, being a pear-shaped woman is a good thing.**

WAIST MEASUREMENT

It's not really weight or total body fat that's linked to ill health—it's *where* that fat lies in the body that's crucial. From a health perspective, being a pear-shaped woman is a good thing. Some of you may love your shape, others may hate it, but take heart that the fat stored on your thighs and bottom does not affect your heart or increase your risk of diabetes. (If you want to keep looking your best, you can certainly work on reducing the amount of fat stored, and on building strength and tone in your upper body to balance your shape.) It's the apple-shaped women among us who really must take action for the sake of their health. Fat around your mid-section is an indication of lots of fat around your internal organs, which is the most damaging. Research has shown that a simple waist measurement is a far stronger indicator of risk of major chronic diseases than weight or BMI. Besides, who among us is not interested in a flatter, leaner midriff? This area of the body is one of our most common problem areas. Having babies and going through menopause are both likely to increase fat around the middle so monitoring your waist measurement is a really good indicator of progress.

Regardless of your height, the medical cut-off points for waist measurement are the same. If your waist is

- **less than 80 centimetres** you're right where you want to be, at least from a health perspective
- **between 80 and 88** you have an increased risk and should lose some mid-section fat
- **greater than 88 centimetres** you seriously need to lose body fat.

Wherever you are on this scale, be realistic. If your waist is currently 120 centimetres there is no point in setting an 80 centimetres waist as your goal. You might achieve it one day, but having such a long-term goal will only demoralise you. Instead, set monthly goals of perhaps 2 centimetres' change; your ultimate aim might be to get down to 110 centimetres. Imagine how fantastic you'll feel to achieve it—that's an 8 per cent change in your waist! Then you can set a new target.

Waisting away

The beauty of a waist measurement is that it is easy to do—you just need a tape measure. You can do it at home and if you see a reduction you can be assured that you are losing body fat. Do take care to measure in the same point each time. Technically, it should be the mid-way point between the top of your hipbone and your lower rib. Most women find it easier to measure either directly around the belly button, or simply around the narrowest point (for hour-glass-shaped women), and this is fine too.

Day-to-day fluctuations in your waist measurement are not changes in fat. Fat takes some time to burn. These changes are likely to be fluid and gas changes in your gut. Many women are plagued with bloating and other gut symptoms. There is no point in measuring your waist daily or weekly. A once-a-month measurement is quite sufficient and more likely to show real change. If you do have major bloating problems see your doctor or dietitian for advice.

OTHER BODY MEASUREMENTS

You can use your tape measure on a number of different areas of your body and this is one of the best means of assessing change. It is important to make sure you measure in the same spot each time, which can be tricky. The best way to do this for limbs is to measure the exact halfway point. For example, if your goal is to lose fat from your thighs, monitor your progress via thigh circumference. First, measure the distance from your groin to your knee, mark the halfway point with a pen and then measure your thigh circumference in line with the mark. Then you'll build an accurate picture of your progress. You can do the same thing for your calves and your upper arms. Around your chest you can measure under or directly around the bust, just as if you were being measured for a bra.

FITNESS

Fitness instructors use any number of different tests to measure your fitness. If you choose the option of either joining a gym or working with a personal trainer you can have them monitor your progress in all aspects of your fitness including cardio, strength and flexibility.

For those who don't want to go that far, you can monitor yourself in these more rudimentary ways (accurate enough to serve the purpose).

Cardio fitness Measure how far you can run, cycle, swim or row. Or if you have the necessary monitoring gizmo to give you speeds along the way, you can use your average speed. This kind of monitoring can fit into your weekly and monthly goals.

There are some great internet tools to assist you with this. For example, Nike have a running website that allows you to track your runs. All you need is their little device that fits in your running shoe and an MP3 player. (You can even download songs and whole workouts.) Once you have completed your run, you hook up your MP3 player and log on to the site. Your run information is downloaded and added to your file. You can then compare every run you do. For someone like me who loves facts and figures, it's a

> **Find what works for you—the only thing for certain is that if you monitor nothing, nothing will change.**

great motivation tool. Of course, others might find this overkill. Do some research and look for a program that works for you.

Strength If you are weight training, keep a log of the weights you use for each exercise. This is a simple means of setting yourself goals and monitoring when you reach them. If you are doing resistance exercises on your own then do a check of how many pushups or situps you can perform. Set a time limit (for example, 1 minute) if you're getting good at them.

Flexibility The classic test is a 'sit and reach' test where you sit on the floor with your legs extended straight in front of you and reach forward with your fingers and see how far you can reach. This really only tests your hip joint flexibility, but since so many of us have tight hamstrings and lower backs, it is still worth doing. For a more comprehensive flexibility test compare your progress in a regular stretch, yoga or balance-style class.

OTHER WAYS TO KEEP TRACK

It's harder to monitor progress towards less tangible goals such as eating more healthily or improving your skin. This is where creative goal-setting using the SMART principles comes in. If you have been specific in setting your goal, you will be able to monitor whether or not you have achieved it. You could perhaps keep a checklist of your goals and tick the box when you have achieved it. This chart serves then as a longer term monitoring tool. It really depends on the type of person you are and the degree of structure you need to make things happen. Some will like to keep to a few handwritten notes in their diary each week, while others will want to set up their own documents and charts on the computer. Find what works for you—the only thing for certain is that if you monitor nothing, nothing will change.

Inner health, outer beauty at a glance

FOOD CHOICE

✳ **Nice and natural** Evaluate food on how close it is to its natural state and not on its fat or carbohydrate content.

✳ **Trust in tradition** Choose traditional tried-and-tested foods over modern processed commercial foods.

✳ **Be an ethical eater** Consume local seasonal produce, fair-trade products and free-range or organic products where possible.

✳ **Release your inner chef** Get into your kitchen and cook and prepare more of your own meals.

✳ **Home cooking rules** When you do have a night off, choose food as close to home cooked as possible. Small takeaway shops serving traditional food are usually much better than the large commercial chains.

✳ **Embrace the ideas** Take from all three ideologies—hedonism (pleasure), nutritionism (health) and spirituality (ethics)—when choosing what and how to eat. The pleasure

of food, the cultural, traditional and social aspects of eating and the sharing of food are just as important as the nutritional factors.

✳ **Not so full-on** Adopt the Okinawan's 'Eat till 80 per cent full' rule.

THOUGHT AND ACTION

✳ **The body talks** Listen to your body and not your environment in choosing when, what and how much to eat.

✳ **Nurture it** Try to have a positive, healthy relationship with food.

✳ **Diet no more** Don't diet—make changes to your eating habits that you can follow forever.

✳ **Not guilty** Stop feeling guilty after eating certain foods. What's done is done—just move on.

✳ **Get good habits** Practise good eating habits such as eating only at the table, and taking your time to savour and enjoy each meal.

* **Emotions in motion** Recognise when you are eating or drinking to quench emotion and develop alternative outlets.

* **Respect yourself** Build good self-esteem and make an effort with your appearance. When you feel good you'll want to eat well and move more.

* **Let there be moral support** Surround yourself with good role models who encourage and inspire you.

CHANGE IN MOTION

* **Get moving** Be an active person who jumps at the chance to move. Develop active behaviours and reduce sedentary ones.

* **Get intense** Build regular bouts of more intense exercise into your week.

* **The joy of movement** Do exercise you enjoy, but recognise that you must expend effort to reap the rewards.

* **Get real** You get the body you are prepared to work for. Don't set unreasonable, unattainable goals.

* **Take control** Exercise should enhance your life, not run your life.

* **Less of the obsess** In a healthy non-emotional way, monitor the changes to your body over time (don't obsess). Small gains are easy to act on with small changes.

* **Under construction** Consider diet and lifestyle change as a work in progress. No one is perfect all of the time.

143

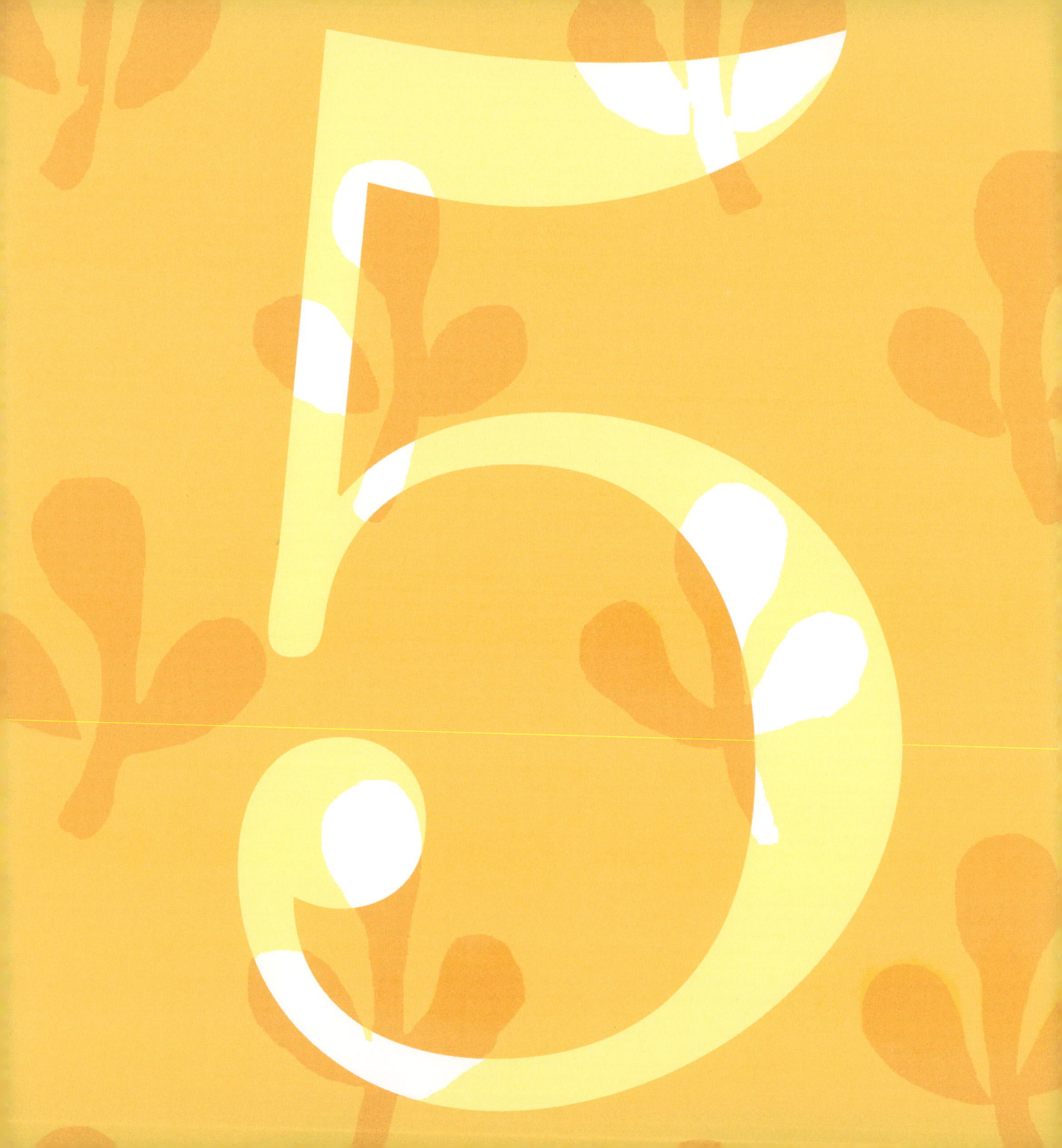

Recipes for life

"Stop thinking and think
and think

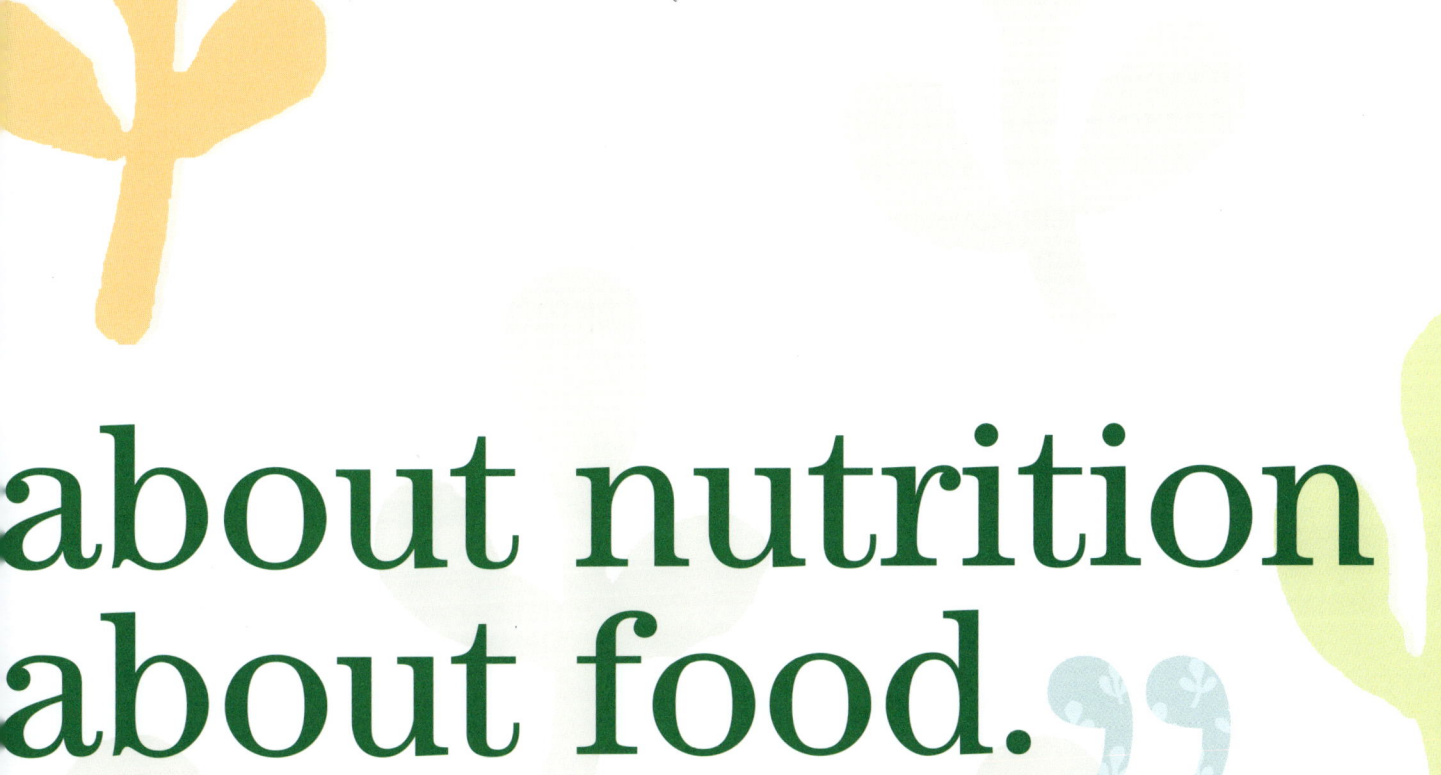

about nutrition
about food. "

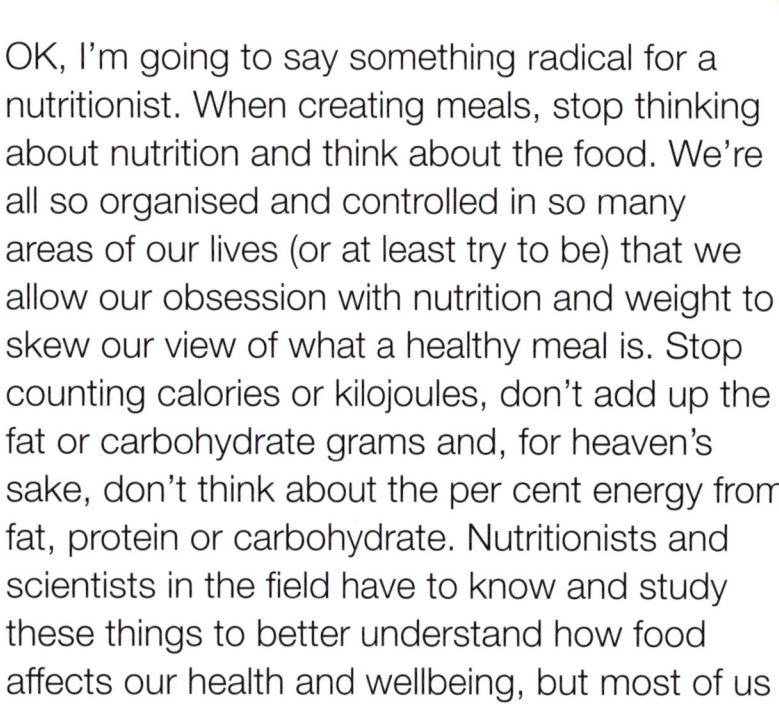
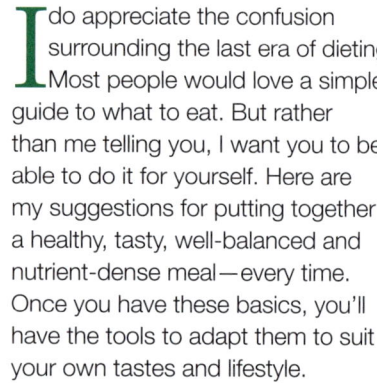

OK, I'm going to say something radical for a nutritionist. When creating meals, stop thinking about nutrition and think about the food. We're all so organised and controlled in so many areas of our lives (or at least try to be) that we allow our obsession with nutrition and weight to skew our view of what a healthy meal is. Stop counting calories or kilojoules, don't add up the fat or carbohydrate grams and, for heaven's sake, don't think about the per cent energy from fat, protein or carbohydrate. Nutritionists and scientists in the field have to know and study these things to better understand how food affects our health and wellbeing, but most of us really don't need such accurate information to create healthy meals.

I do appreciate the confusion surrounding the last era of dieting. Most people would love a simple guide to what to eat. But rather than me telling you, I want you to be able to do it for yourself. Here are my suggestions for putting together a healthy, tasty, well-balanced and nutrient-dense meal—every time. Once you have these basics, you'll have the tools to adapt them to suit your own tastes and lifestyle.

First up, fill half your plate with veggies (and/or fruit depending on the meal). They'll provide volume and filling power for not many kilojoules. They're packed with the nutrients, fibre and phytochemicals our bodies require and are definitely worthy of the biggest space on the plate.

I know I just said don't think about the big macronutrients—fat, carbohydrate and protein—but it does help to use these terms to broadly categorise foods into groups. We need sources of all three in our diet and so the second half of the plate is split between them. While I by no means adhere to the strict low-fat message of the past couple of decades, fat is energy-dense stuff and we don't need

much of it. It does provide important nutrients, it is necessary to absorb certain antioxidants (including beta-carotene) and just as importantly it tastes good. Taking all these factors into account, it gets a smaller, but no less important, slice of the pie. A drizzle of olive oil, some mashed avocado, a sprinkle of nuts or a dollop of hummus are all great, healthy examples.

The remaining space is split between our carbs and proteins. Almost all carbs—breads, pasta, grains and legumes—provide some protein, many very good levels of protein, so I prefer to call them carb-rich foods rather than carbs. Animal sources of protein almost always provide significant levels of

fat so you can see there is also a crossover here. While plant sources of protein almost always provide carbohydrates and varying levels of fat, I prefer to call them protein-rich foods. The idea of classifying foods is just to be able to pull together a meal that is varied, therefore giving a broad range of nutrients without too much of any one thing. Finally, from every food group we want to be sure to choose the best-quality foods that we can. The key yet again is balance.

"From every food group we want to be sure to choose the best-quality foods that we can."

The middle line

The lines between the fat-rich, carb-rich and protein-rich foods are not immutable. The most important factor on your plate is the middle line, ensuring you half-fill the plate with veggies and/or fruit. The remaining half is more flexible, depending on what you're having, your likes and dislikes, where you are and what you'll have for other meals during the day. For example, if you have just finished a pretty tough cardio workout you'll probably want a few extra carbs to restock your body's stores. Or you may feel better on a higher protein diet with fewer grain foods. Or perhaps you had a large steak while you were out for lunch and feel like a lighter vegetarian supper (this is likely to have more carb-rich foods and fewer protein-rich ones). All these options are fine.

 **Think about the meals you eat regularly. See if they fit these suggestions, or could be adapted to fit. You may find you are eating fairly healthy foods, but may have to readjust the portion sizes of each food group.**

The two most important factors are:

1 Fill half the plate with veggies and/or fruit

2 Choose fresh, natural, good-quality foods from several different food groups. For example:

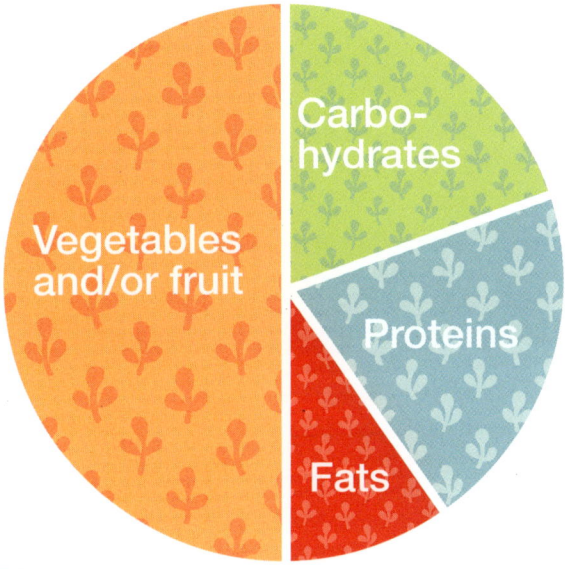

Breakfast
- blueberries, strawberries, banana and peach (fruit)
- muesli (carbs)
- low-fat milk and natural yoghurt (protein)
- nuts and seeds (fat)

Lunch
- rocket, tomato, beetroot, carrot, sprouts (veggies)
- wholegrain mountain bread wrap (carbs)
- chicken breast (protein)
- hummus (fat)

Dinner
- salad greens, capsicum, tomatoes, cucumber, mango (fruit and veggies)
- fish fillet (protein)
- freekeh and corn salad (carbs)
- avocado and olive oil (fat)

- broccoli, green beans and mushrooms (veggies)
- kangaroo fillet (protein)
- sweet potato wedges (carbs)
- camellia tea oil (fat)

This goes with that...

Carbohydrate-rich foods

Whole grains, corn, starchy vegetables, legumes

BEST CHOICES

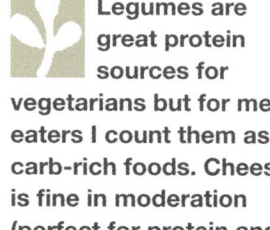 **Legumes are great protein sources for vegetarians but for meat eaters I count them as carb-rich foods. Cheese is fine in moderation (perfect for protein and calcium but high in saturated fat).**

- rolled oats
- brown rice
- quinoa
- freekeh
- barley
- pasta
- Asian noodles (not instant flavoured varieties)
- wholegrain low GI breakfast cereals
- wholegrain low GI bread
- whole corn (fresh, frozen or canned)
- sweet potatoes, yam or taro, small waxy potatoes
- lentils, dried beans (canned is fine) and peas

Protein-rich foods

Meat, poultry, fish, seafood, eggs, dairy, tofu and tempeh

BEST CHOICES
- lean cuts of meat (grass-fed, free-range, hormone- and antibiotic-free)
- wild meats (such as kangaroo or venison)
- sustainable fish
- seafood (mussels, oysters, prawns, octopus, squid)
- free-range or organic eggs
- low-fat milk
- natural yoghurt
- tofu
- tempeh

Fat-rich foods

Oils, butter, margarine, nuts, seeds and avocado

BEST CHOICES
- nuts, seeds and oils extracted from them (cold-pressed oils are best quality)
- nut butters (unadulterated)
- avocado and avocado oil
- olives and olive oil
- camellia tea oil
- coconut oil

Margarines don't conform to my rule to eat things as close as possible to nature. Butter is high in saturated fat, but I prefer to use a little of this than a manufactured processed margarine. It's a personal choice. If you have high cholesterol you'd be best to skip the butter completely.

Real meal deals

I know how hard it can be to think about meals week in, week out, whether you are cooking for yourself or for a family. It is no wonder there has been such a rise in the sales of pre-prepared meals and takeaway. There is nothing wrong with using these services once or twice a week when you really can't summon up the energy to cook, or when there is truly nothing in the fridge—it happens to us all. But remember: make your choices carefully. However, to truly embrace our new philosophies and reclaim your natural beauty, you have to get into your kitchen and be in control of more of your own meals. With a little planning and a few kitchen skills you'll discover that it's really not that hard. For those of you who already cook regularly I hope I can give you a few new ideas and alert you to changes you can make to attune your cooking and meals to virbrant health. If you're worried that all this healthy eating will cost more, think again. If you actually add up how much you spend on takeaway, you're probably in for a shock. There is no doubt that cooking at home from the raw ingredients is infinitely cheaper, particularly with good planning and very little food wastage. For example, see our tips for buying a whole chicken and producing several meals from that one purchase. Perhaps you could treat yourself to a new haircut, a facial or a new outfit with all the money you save!

We are bombarded with messages about cooking that are not true, for example: 'I don't have time to cook.'

Really? A fabulous meal can be knocked up in 20 minutes, faster than it would take you to drive to the takeaway shop. Jamie Oliver famously cooked a pizza from scratch faster than the deliveryman could get one to him while on stage. Cooking needn't take all afternoon in the kitchen, with the right skills and know-how.

We are also led to believe that cooking is a chore and that we have better things to do with our time. Well, I believe our bodies deserve more than a microwave meal or greasy takeaway. Many of you seem to agree with me. Of the women who took part in my survey, 76 per cent said they liked to cook and a further 21 per cent said they liked to cook sometimes. When asked if they felt cooking was a chore, 31 cent said no, only 4 per cent said yes and the remaining 65 per cent admitted it was sometimes.

The better skills and sassy meal ideas you have, the less of a chore cooking becomes. The trick is to cook quickly and with flair. If you hate to cook, or think you can't, reset your thinking. Cooking and preparing food should be a basic daily activity. After all, our mothers, grandmothers and great-grandmothers, all the way back to hunter–gatherer days, have gathered and prepared food to nourish themselves and their family. Make the most of it—and you just might find you enjoy it. The reward is immediate in the taste of the food and in the way that you feel after a superbly healthy meal.

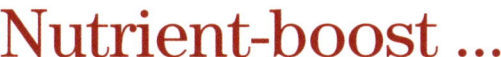

Nutrient-boost ...

Your breakfast ...

Muesli with milk and a sliced strawberry or two

Better breakfast

Reduce the muesli portion, increase the fruit substantially and add some natural yoghurt to boost the protein. *Bonus*: If you're trying to lose weight this also reduces kilojoules and increases the satiety factor.

Your lunch ...

Ham and cheese sandwich on white or brown bread

Better lunch

Change the type of bread to a spelt sourdough, or simply a nice wholegrain loaf, add a whole host of veggies (lettuce, beetroot, tomato, cucumber, grated carrot) and some mashed avocado for good fat and flavour. Ham is very salty and contains preservatives; cheese is OK now and again. A better choice would be some lean meat, chicken or canned fish.

Your dinner ...

Meat and two veg, one of these being potatoes

Better dinner

Reduce the meat portion (to the size of the palm of your hand), swap the potatoes for more nutritious and lower GI sweet potato, and give a serious boost to the veggies in volume and colourful variety. Stir-fry them with garlic, ginger and a squeeze of lemon juice. *Bonus*: The whole meal is much more interesting and steps up nutritionally. When you've really enjoyed such a dinner you will feel less inclined to raid the pantry for a little treat later in the evening.

SAMMIE CORYTON
To inspire you in the kitchen I recruited London-based chef and all-round gorgeous girl Sammie Coryton to help me create meal ideas and recipes. The key word here is 'idea' as the recipes aren't rigidly fixed. If you don't have one or two ingredients, feel free to replace them with something else—in fact, we encourage it! It will help boost your creativity. We want you to get into your kitchen and experiment. If you are a novice cook, by all means try the recipes as they are written. As you get more confident we hope you will develop your own ideas or start with one of ours and then diversify into your own. Nothing here is cordon bleu level; everything is for the home cook like you or me. Happy cooking!

Breakfast

I don't really go with the 'breakfast is the most important meal of the day' nor the idea that we should eat 'like a king' at breakfast. All meals are important nutritionally and the reality of most of our lives is that dinner tends to be when we have the time to relax and enjoy a larger meal. Some people are also not big breakfast eaters and that is fine. However, breakfast does affect us physically and biologically as it breaks the longest time without incoming food that our body usually has, that is overnight. So what you choose affects your blood sugar and insulin levels much more than at later meals. The good news is that breakfast is not hard to get right.

Steer clear of most breakfast cereals—they are processed carbs (and therefore usually high GI) with a few vitamins and minerals added back in, often with a good whack of sugar and salt as well. Instead go for fruit, whole grains, low-GI cereals, yoghurt or a hot brekkie of eggs with plenty of veggies.

SUPER-EASY MUESLI AND FRUIT

Store-bought natural muesli (look for one with no added sugar or salt), softened with some low-fat milk or a non-dairy alternative (soy drink, rice/oat milk, fruit juice), topped with a generous selection of fresh fruit (berries, sliced banana, diced mango) and a dollop of natural yoghurt.

OR

Soak natural muesli or just plain rolled oats in apple juice overnight in the fridge. Sometimes I also add a handful of sultanas or other dried fruit to the overnight mix. In the morning stir through some natural yoghurt and top with fresh or dried fruit and a sprinkling of whatever nuts and seeds you have in the pantry.

JOANNA'S DIY MUESLI

This is different every time I make it, so follow the idea here rather than the recipe. All you have to do is buy a variety of different nuts, seeds and dried fruit, and mix them with rolled oats in a large bowl. Transfer to an airtight container and it will last you at least a couple of weeks. The advantage is you can add your own favourite ingredients and avoid those you don't like in the shop-bought versions. Try these ingredient ideas:

- Rolled oats, barley, spelt or other cereal grains

- Sultanas, raisins, currants, dried apricots, dried apple, dried figs (organic or those that state no preservatives used are best, otherwise they will contain sulphite preservatives)

- Almonds, macadamias, cashews, Brazil nuts, walnuts, hazelnuts, sunflower seeds, peptitas—they are nicer roasted which you can do yourself in a hot oven for a few minutes, or buy them roasted but without added salt

Supercharge

Having grown up in Scotland, oats have always been a staple food in my life and rightfully so. Oats are one of the best-known foods to help reduce cholesterol. They're rich in soluble fibre, they have a low GI and are relatively high in protein for a grain. They also provide many other vitamins and minerals, most notably the anti-ageing, disease-fighting antioxidant vitamin E—a 100 gram serve of oats in the morning provides 20 per cent of the vitamin E us girls need for the day.

TANGY NUTTY TOAST AND FRUIT

Start with a bowl of fruit salad topped with a dollop of natural yoghurt. (If you are in a rush, fruit salad direct from a carton or tub, soaked in fruit juice not syrup, is fine, just not as tasty as fresh). Follow this with my version of the very American peanut butter and jelly sandwich, but much healthier. Toast a slice of good-quality sourdough or wholegrain bread and top with nut butter (I like the ABC spread—a blend of almonds, Brazil nuts and cashew nuts) and top with pure orange fruit spread. A sweeter alternative is to use honey in place of the fruit spread.

CAN'T STOMACH BREAKFAST?

For non-breakfast eaters your best bet is to go liquid—smoothies are hard to beat. Basically blitz together low-fat milk (or a dairy alternative such as soy, rice or oat milk) with whatever fresh fruit you have and a good dollop of natural yoghurt. Add some wheat germ or oat bran for fibre if you have it in your pantry, but to be honest I rarely bother—I prefer to get my fibre elsewhere.

EGGS OVER EASY

Eggs are hard to beat for breakfast and nutritionally they are a fabulous food providing numerous micronutrients. In summer I love to poach them and serve on a slice of rye sourdough with any combination of sliced smoked salmon, sliced avocado, wilted spinach, a fresh vine-ripened tomato and a sliced field mushroom sautéed in olive oil.

OR

I simply boil them until gooey (4 minutes for a runny yolk, 5 minutes for soft and gooey) and serve them with sourdough toast 'soldiers'. You can have a little butter if you like or I prefer to use a little reduced-fat cream cheese. Follow up with half a ruby red grapefruit and a glass of fruit and veg juice—V8 brand juices are convenient and absolutely fine. If you have a juicer, make your own.

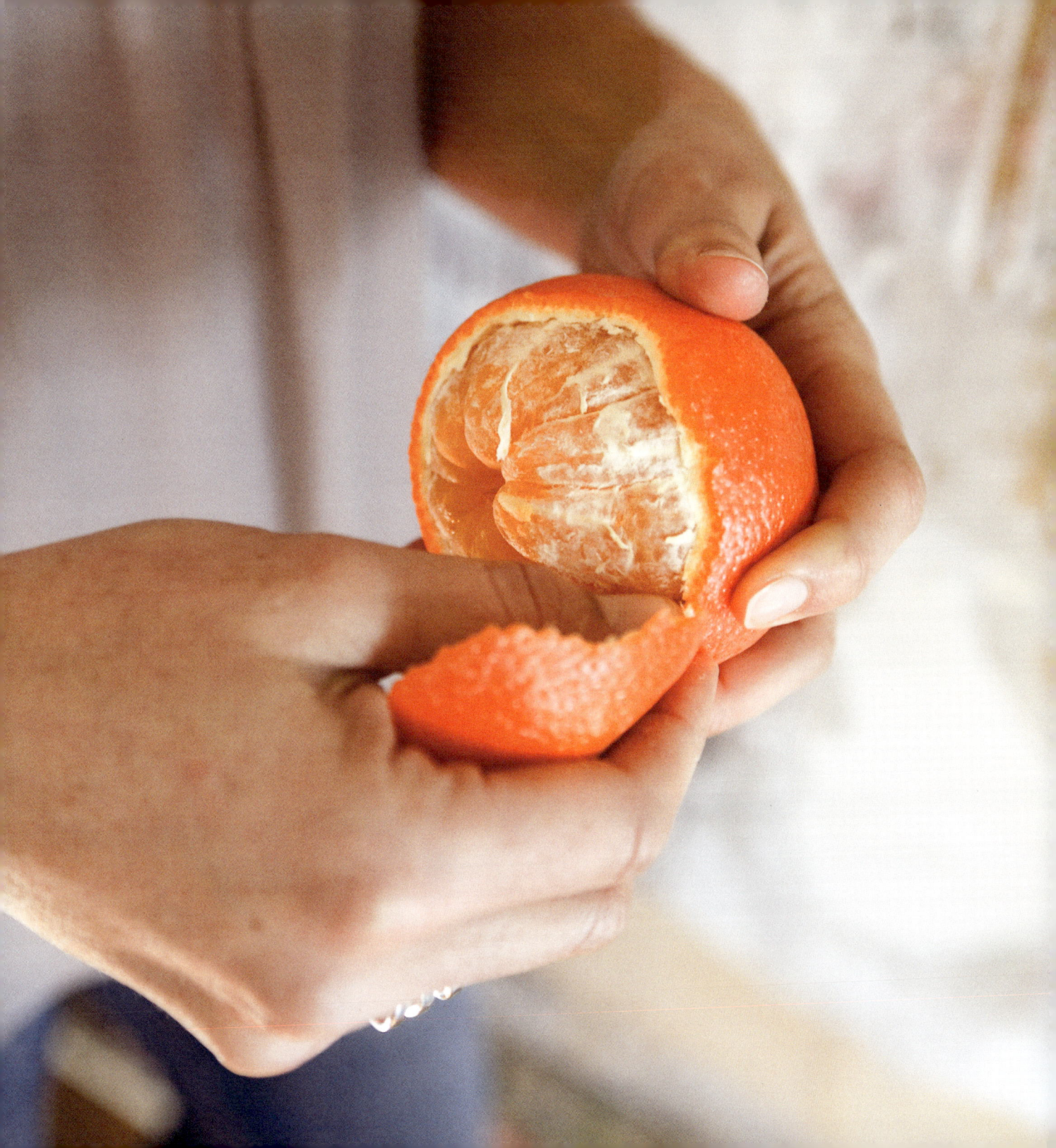

Tropical fruit salad with toasted nut and seed topping

The nut and seed mixture can be made using any combination you like or have in the pantry. Once you've completed steps 1 to 4 you can store the mixture in an airtight jar. You should then have enough for about two weeks' worth of breakfasts with minimal effort involved.

Level of effort: 2
Prep time: 15 minutes
Cook time: 10 minutes
Serves 6

2 tablespoons pepitas
2 tablespoons sunflower seeds
¼ cup sesame seeds
2 tablespoons shredded coconut
⅓ cup hazelnuts, toasted, chopped
⅓ cup pecans, toasted, chopped
⅓ cup (80ml) agave nectar

Selection of ripe tropical
    fruit (pineapple, mango,
    passionfruit, kiwifruit, dragon
    fruit, bananas)
Strawberries, hulled and chopped
Natural sheep's milk yoghurt
    (wonderfully rich and creamy)

Preheat oven to 180°C (160°C fan-forced).

Place nuts and seeds on a baking tray and roast in preheated oven 5 minutes, stirring once or twice until golden brown.

Drizzle agave nectar over the toasted nuts and seeds and return to the oven for a further 2–3 minutes or until starting to smell nice and toasty.

Remove seed mixture from the oven and set aside to cool.

Make fruit salad by combining ingredients in a large bowl. Stir gently to combine.

Divide fruit among bowls and top each serving with a generous dollop of yoghurt and a handful of the toasted cool nut and seed mixture.

Supercharge

Agave nectar is a natural sweetener produced from the succulent agave plant that grows in the US and tropical America. You can buy it in health food stores and some good grocers. It has a low GI, meaning the sugars are slowly absorbed and help you to keep your blood sugar levels steady.

Apple and coconut Bircher muesli with prune and apple compote

I love Bircher muesli and for those who think regular muesli is better suited to horses, I promise this style will win you over! The compote is a real nutritional winner with the combination of antioxidant-rich and fibre-rich apples and prunes. The compote can be made in advance and can be kept in the fridge for several days. Then all you have to remember is to do step 1 before you go to bed and the level of morning effort drops to a 1.

Level of effort: 2
Prep time: 20 minutes (plus overnight soaking)
Cook time: 5 minutes
Serves: 6–8 (recipe can be halved)

3 cups rolled oats
1 cup toasted sunflower seeds
1 cup toasted flaked or shredded coconut
1 apple, grated (unpeeled)

1½ cups (375ml) natural unsweetened apple juice
1½ cups (375ml) milk

1 cup seeded prunes, chopped
3 large apples, peeled, seeded, chopped
2 tablespoons lemon juice

To serve
Natural yoghurt, the compote and chopped toasted hazelnuts

For the Bircher muesli: Combine all dry ingredients in a large bowl. Add apple juice and milk and stir well. Cover and refrigerate overnight.

Make the compote by combining prunes, apples and juice in a small saucepan. Place over a low heat and cover until the apples start to release their juices before bringing to a boil and simmering for 2 minutes. Remove from the heat and cool.

To serve, stir 2 tablespoons natural yoghurt into each serving. Add extra milk if desired and top with the compote and hazelnuts.

Supercharge

Prunes might be most famous for their ability to get your bowels moving, but let's not underestimate the importance of that! They are also little nutrition bombs—the nutrients found in plums, including the antioxidants, are concentrated in prunes. Furthermore, they have a low GI, making them an ideal addition to breakfast and to eat on their own as a convenient snack.

Joanna's fruity porridge with maple syrup

Although many of the more summery ideas also work in winter, there are some mornings when you just want something warming and hearty. You can't beat the Scot out of me and so porridge is my overwhelming favourite. However, I've grown fond of the Aussie fruity versions and so here is my favourite take, after much experimentation with various combinations.

Combine 1 cup of rolled oats and 2 cups of water in a pan. Bring to the boil and reduce the heat to simmer for 10 minutes or so, stirring a few times along the way. (This quantity feeds me and my two kids—adjust to suit your requirements). Serve in bowls topped with fresh fruit in season, some warmed low-fat milk or soy drink and a drizzle of maple syrup (or honey if you prefer).

You can reduce the cooking time further by soaking the oats overnight in the fridge, or even for about 20 minutes in the morning while you have your shower. Cook for 5 minutes and you're ready to eat.

OR

Add a few frozen packet berries to the porridge mixture in the last few minutes of cooking. Don't let the resultant colour put you off—my kids call it 'purple porridge' and the taste is delicious. Sliced banana also works well added during cooking.

OR

Try making a porridge using other grains such as quinoa, barley or spelt. I buy a Finnish porridge mixture at my local health food store, which contains a mix of rolled oats, rye, barley and spelt. It makes a wonderfully nutty, hearty porridge. Perfect for a cold winter morning.

French toast with berry compote

This recipe tastes truly decadent but, providing you use good-quality bread, it is gloriously healthy. The sweetness comes from maple syrup, one of nature's delicious gifts. Be sure to buy pure maple syrup and not the cheaper imitation maple-flavoured syrup (the latter is refined, made in a factory and has a high GI, while the real thing is collected direct from Canadian maple trees and has a low GI).

Level of effort: 1
Prep time: 15 minutes
Cook time: 15 minutes
Serves 4

½ cup (125ml) low-fat milk
2 free-range eggs, lightly beaten
2 tablespoons maple syrup
½ teaspoon ground cinnamon
6 thick slices sourdough bread

300g mixed frozen berries
¼ cup (60ml) orange juice
2 tablespoons maple syrup

Combine milk, eggs, maple syrup and cinnamon in a large bowl. Dip bread slices into mixture and press down to absorb egg mixture. Leave to soak in mixture for 5 minutes.

Combine berries, orange juice and maple syrup in a small saucepan over a medium heat. Simmer 5 minutes until berries soften and juices run.

Heat a non-stick frying pan over a high heat. Spray lightly with cooking oil spray or a tiny amount of olive oil. Fry drained bread slices 3 minutes or until crisp and golden; transfer to a plate lined with absorbent paper. Cut bread slices in half and serve with the warm berries.

Supercharge

Berries are hard to beat for total antioxidant power, principally from the anthocyanins, which give them their glorious red and purple colour. They're also rich in vitamin C, essential for collagen production and young-looking skin. Some berries have antibacterial qualities that help prevent infections that plague some women, such as cystitis. Fresh berries can be expensive when they're not in season. The solution is to buy frozen— convenient, available and the nutrients are preserved.

Eggs with cucumber, avocado, mint and yoghurt

Level of effort: 2
Prep time: 15 minutes
Cook time: 5 minutes
Serves 4

1 Lebanese cucumber
½ lemon
1 small avocado, chopped
    coarsely
½ cup mint leaves
1 cup plain natural yoghurt
pinch salt
paprika

1 tablespoon olive oil
4 organic free-range eggs
4 slices sourdough bread
3 vine-ripened tomatoes, chopped
    coarsely, optional
freshly ground black pepper

Using a vegetable peeler, half peel the cucumber so that the skin becomes striped. Cut in half lengthways and scoop out the seeds. Cut into 5mm slices on the diagonal.

Combine cucumber slices with half the lemon juice, the avocado and the mint leaves.

Combine yoghurt with the salt and set aside.

Heat a griddle pan and toast the sourdough until golden. Meanwhile, heat a large frying pan and add the oil. Cook eggs for 3 minutes so that the white has set but the yolks are still runny.

Serve eggs on the sourdough toast with the cucumber and avocado salad and the tomatoes on the side and a dollop of yoghurt on top. Sprinkle with paprika and freshly ground black pepper.

Supercharge

The humble egg, as we've always known, provides many essential nutrients. But an Australian study (2007) elevates it to lofty nutritional heights. Eggs were found to be much higher in essential long-chain omega-3 fats than previously thought, making them particularly good for anyone who doesn't eat fish and a great omega boost for the rest of us. Eggs were also found to be a good source of iodine, a mineral often low in Australian diets. Iodine is necessary for proper thyroid function, and thus metabolism, and a good iodine intake during pregnancy is particularly important (iodine deficiency can cause miscarriage, stillbirth or mental impairment in the baby). Eggs for breakfast can even curb morning hunger so you tend to eat less for the rest of the day. Gone are the days of limiting our eggs based on incorrect beliefs about their effect on cholesterol. It looks like eggs are in, in, in!

Poached eggs on spiced sweet potato cakes

Level of effort: 2
Prep time: 10 minutes
Cook time: 15 minutes
Serves 4

½ teaspoon black mustard seeds
1 teaspoon cumin seeds
½ teaspoon coriander seeds
1 medium sweet potato, peeled, grated
2 tablespoons finely chopped fresh coriander
½ teaspoon dried chilli flakes
pinch sea salt
1 egg
1 tablespoon olive oil

2 teaspoons white wine vinegar
4 eggs
coriander sprigs

Dry-fry mustard, cumin and coriander seeds until lightly fragrant. Transfer to a pestle and mortar and crush coarsely.

Combine in a large bowl with the sweet potato, coriander, chilli flakes, salt and egg and mix until well combined.

Heat olive oil in a large frying pan and add spoonfuls of the sweet potato mixture, pressing them out to form a patty, no thicker than 1.5 cm. Fry 3–4 minutes each side until the potato cakes are golden on both sides and cooked through. Transfer to a baking tray and keep warm in a low oven while you poach the eggs.

Place a deep frying pan that is half full of water on to boil. Once it is simmering add the vinegar and reduce the heat so that the bubbles are just moving in the barely simmering water. One by one, crack the eggs into the simmering water and cook for about 4 minutes each until the whites are set and the yolk still runny.

Remove the eggs from the water with a slotted spoon and drain on absorbent paper.

Arrange two potato cakes on each serving plate and top them with a poached egg. Garnish with freshly cracked black pepper and some sprigs of coriander. A drizzle of sweet chilli sauce would be a delicious accompaniment.

Baked eggs en cocotte with leeks, peas and onions

Level of effort: 2
Prep time: 10 minutes
Cook time: 25 minutes
Serves 6

1 tablespoon olive oil
1 small onion, chopped finely
1 small leek, sliced thinly
½ cup peas, frozen or fresh
1 tablespoon flat-leaf parsley,
    shredded
1 clove garlic, halved
6 eggs
smoked paprika, optional
sourdough toast, cut into soldiers
    to serve

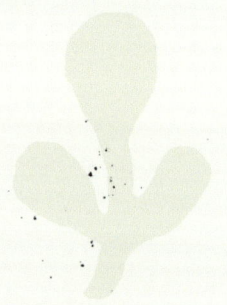 **You need six ramekin dishes for this recipe.**

Preheat oven to 200°C (180°C fan-forced).

Heat half of the olive oil in a frying pan and cook onion and leek until softened and translucent.

Add peas and cook a further minute or two until they are tender.

Season the mixture with salt and pepper and stir in the parsley.

Rub cut side of the garlic clove around the inside of the lightly greased ramekins. Divide the pea and leek mixture among the ramekins.

Crack an egg into each ramekin over the top of the vegetables and sprinkle each one with a little paprika, and salt and pepper if desired.

Transfer ramekins to the preheated oven (putting them on a baking tray makes removing them much easier). Cook 12–15 minutes or until egg whites are set and yolks are still runny.

Serve with sourdough soldiers.

Supercharge
Onions, garlic and leeks are all part of the *Allium* family of vegetables. They provide a number of powerful antioxidants that have earned them 'superfood' status, including sulphur compounds shown to prevent tumour growth in research studies. They are also great for gut health. And if your gut functions well, there is a knock-on effect on how you look and how you feel.

Homemade baked beans

Canned supermarket baked beans are fine as a pantry standby (the reduced-salt variety) but homemade baked beans are indescribably better. Don't be put off by the cooking and soaking time, as the actual cooking time is only 20 minutes. Try making them on the weekend when you have more time and they will keep in the fridge for several days. I also like to freeze one to two extra batches.

Level of effort: 3

Prep time: 20 minutes + 2 hours soaking time

Cooking time: 2 hours

Serves 6

500g dried navy beans or cannellini beans

2 tablespoons olive oil

1 large onion, diced

3 cloves garlic, chopped

100g pancetta, chopped into lardons (or cubed, if easier), optional

700g bottle passata (thick tomato sauce)

¼ cup treacle

2 tablespoons maple syrup

2 tablespoons Worcestershire sauce

1 tablespoon apple cider vinegar

2 bay leaves

1 tablespoon dry English mustard

¼ teaspoon ground cloves

¼ teaspoon smoked paprika*

sea salt and freshly ground black pepper

2 cups (500ml) chicken stock

Soak beans overnight in plenty of cold water.

The following day, drain and rinse the beans and boil them in plenty of clean water for up to 1½ hours until they are tender and softened.

Preheat the oven to 160°C (140°C fan-forced). If using canned beans no soaking or cooking is needed but use a hotter oven of 180°C.

Heat oil in a large enamelled cast-iron casserole. Sauté onion, garlic and pancetta (if using) until lightly browned and the fat has run from the pancetta.

Add the remaining ingredients, including the beans, and bring to the boil.

Cover and bake casserole in preheated oven for 2 hours (1 hour for canned beans).

Remove bay leaves before serving with a generous bunch of wilted spinach and a grilled vine-ripened tomato. They are also delicious topped with a poached egg.

 Smoked paprika is available from delicatessens and gourmet food stores.

Ten foods for radiant skin, strong nails and luscious locks

1

Salmon Oily fish such as salmon are fabulously rich in the essential omega-3 fats. These reduce inflammation and provide essential nourishment to the skin. Other oily fish include sardines, mackerel, anchovies and trout. To benefit from oily fish you have to eat it at least twice a week. I also recommend taking an additional daily omega-3 supplement otherwise optimal levels are hard to reach. If you suffer from eczema or psoriasis you should up the dose—there's good scientific backing to show it can help. Oily fish are also one of few food sources of vitamin D, essential for the absorption of calcium to build strong nails.

2

Dark green leafy veggies These are a daily must for maximum anti-ageing power. The darker green the better, because this usually indicates higher levels of antioxidants. These fight the free radicals that damage cells and accelerate ageing of the skin. Beta-carotene, one of these antioxidants, can also form vitamin A in the body, a common ingredient in face creams and an essential nutrient for healthy hair. Feed your skin from the inside out by including leafy greens daily and watch your skin bloom. Spinach, silver beet, kale, rocket, watercress, Asian greens and dark green cabbage varieties all qualify.

3

Mussels and oysters High in protein, good sources of omega-3 fats and the clear front runners for providing zinc, a mineral essential for skin healing and preventing infections. Increased zinc can help acne and other skin conditions, but is also essential for all of us to maintain healthy radiant skin. If you are plagued with dandruff, upping your zinc just might help.

4

Berries They look delectable, they taste divine and they top the charts for antioxidant power. What's not to like about berries? They're also rich in vitamin C, an antioxidant to combat the ageing process, but also necessary for the building of collagen, the protein that gives skin its elasticity and strengthens capillaries to help reduce spider veins and easy bruising.

5 **Nuts and seeds** They provide all the right kinds of fat that nourish our skin and promote shiny healthy hair. They are also rich in the antioxidant vitamin E to combat free-radical damage, which contributes to skin ageing.

6 **Carrots** This humble veggie is one of the richest sources of beta-carotene, which acts both as an antioxidant in its own right and can be made into vitamin A, which repairs and maintains healthy skin.

7 **Tea** Different teas contain different antioxidants, but they all have the potential for anti-ageing benefits. Green tea has even been shown to help rejuvenate skin cells. Tannins in tea can reduce your absorption of minerals in food, however, so try to drink your tea between rather than with meals.

8 **Barley** Australian research has recently shown that a low-GI diet containing whole grains such as barley helps to relieve acne and improve the skin. Barley also provides the antioxidant mineral selenium and good levels of several other vitamins and minerals that play roles in the growth of healthy skin, hair and nails.

9 **Avocado** Arguably the most nutritious food, avocados provide all the right kinds of fat to nourish your skin, numerous vitamins and minerals, and several antioxidants that help to protect your skin from ageing free-radical and sun damage.

10 **Kiwi fruit** We tend to think of citrus fruit as being the best sources of vitamin C, but in fact the plentiful kiwi fruit ranks second only to the more elusive guava. So go green and hairy for extra collagen-boosting vitamin C.

Lunch or light meals

A well-put-together salad is perfect for a summer lunch. Just remember to add some protein-rich food to keep hunger pangs at bay for the afternoon. Live it up—be adventurous with the veggies you add. There's plenty of variety at this time of year.

I never have salad without a great dressing—and it's not just about the taste. You'll eat more salad veggies if they are deliciously dressed, and the oil in the dressing also helps you to absorb the antioxidants and other fat-soluble nutrients in the salad.

CREATE YOUR OWN ... AT THE SALAD BAR

Step up to the salad bar to put together your own perfect salads at home or for your lunch box. These ideas can inspire you at a takeaway salad bar where you can create your own healthy meal on the run. The level of effort is 1 for takeaway or 2 if you make yourself.

Step 1: **CHOOSE** your leaves, the greener the better. Try any type of lettuce, baby English spinach leaves, rocket, snowpea sprouts, watercress, silver beet (remove all white parts and the leaves are delicious raw), beetroot leaves, and fresh herbs (for example, mint, flat-leaf parsley, basil).

Step 2: **ADD** a variety of chopped veggies, the more colourful the better. Try sliced capsicum, whole cherry tomatoes (or sundried), chunks of cucumber, slivers of green onion, corn, grated fresh beetroot, olives, ribbons of carrot, finely shredded red cabbage, blanched green beans, raw peas, or broccoli florets. Some fruits are also delicious in salads—try mango, orange or pink grapefruit segments, pomegranate seeds, diced apple or pear, or diced avocado.

Step 3: **ADD** a protein-rich food, for example cold or hot sliced lean meat, chicken, smoked fish, hard-boiled egg, goat's cheese, feta, marinated tofu, beans, chickpeas or lentils and/or a handful of nuts or seeds.

Step 4: **DRESS** with a delicious dressing made from good-quality oil (choose cold-pressed olive, nut, avocado or camellia tea oil). Basically a 3:1 ratio of oil to vinegar works and you can try different combinations of oils and vinegars. (See our suggestions to follow.)

OPTION Step 5: **ADD** a good quality carb. This is not always necessary and depends on how hungry you are, what you feel like and what exercise you have been doing. Vegetarians who may not have added a protein-rich food should certainly add a grain here to boost the protein at the same time. Choose from low GI wholegrain bread, brown rice, freekeh, quinoa or other cooked whole grain.

Traditional olive oil vinaigrette

My favourite vinaigrette combines quality vinegar and good olive oil. I'm not a fan of pieces of raw garlic in my salads, so I tend to leave the garlic out of the dressing, but instead rub a cut raw garlic clove around the inside of the salad bowl before adding the leaves. This adds the perfect garlicky hint. You can also make the dressing in the salad bowl before adding the leaves. Drizzle the vinegar and oil down the sides of the salad bowl to take up the garlic flavour.

Prep time: 5 minutes
Makes ¾ cup

2 tablespoons white wine vinegar
pinch sugar
pinch of sea salt
1 teaspoon Dijon mustard
freshly ground black pepper
6 tablespoons extra virgin olive oil

Place 2 tablespoons white wine vinegar into a bowl or jug and add a pinch of sugar, pinch of salt and a teaspoon of Dijon mustard.

Whisk lightly until the mustard breaks down and the crystals of sugar and salt have dissolved.

Season with plenty of black pepper. Add the extra virgin olive oil, whisking continuously.

 **This dressing is really versatile. It doesn't matter what kind of acidic base you use (citrus juice, white wine vinegar, balsamic vinegar) and it doesn't even matter if you don't have olive oil. You'll make a good dressing if you get the balance of acid versus oil correct. So, use one part acid for three to four parts oil depending on the strength of your acid. I like to use the acid as my base, and add any flavouring, such as salt, sugar, mustard to that. Oil is not a good solvent and so you will find that the flavours disperse through the dressing more readily if you add them to the acid at the beginning.**

Adding the oil as you whisk helps create a thick, emulsified, traditional vinaigrette. You can also make it in a screw-top jar. Give the ingredients a good shake to get a similar result to whisking.

Avocado oil, orange and hazelnut dressing

As for the traditional vinaigrette, the balance of flavours is all-important. Because orange juice is quite sweet, I like to add a teaspoon of white wine vinegar, but this is optional.

Prep time: 5 minutes

2 tablespoons orange juice
1 teaspoon white wine vinegar
   (optional)
1 teaspoon wholegrain mustard
salt and pepper
1 tablespoon hazelnut oil
5 tablespoons avocado oil

Combine orange juice, vinegar, mustard, salt and pepper in a small bowl. Whisk to combine before gradually adding the oils.

Serve this dressing with a selection of lettuce leaves. It works particularly well if you include something slightly bitter, for example endive and witlof. Adding a handful of toasted hazelnuts and some chopped avocado is great also. This salad is delicious with steamed or grilled chicken or fish.

173

Asian dressing

This dressing must strike a balance between hot, sour, salty and sweet. You should be able to taste all four flavours, one after another. If not, increase the amount of one ingredient at a time until you achieve that balance.

Prep time: 5 minutes

⅓ cup (80ml) lime juice, about 3
    limes
3 teaspoons palm sugar, grated or
    chopped
1 red chilli, seeded, finely chopped
3 teaspoons fish sauce
dash of sesame oil

Combine all ingredients in a screw-top jar, then shake well to combine.

Add a little camellia tea oil if you want to extend the dressing. Serve over plain leaves to liven them up a little or over cooked noodles with chicken, sliced cucumber, halved cherry tomatoes and fresh herbs for a refreshing summer salad. It could also be used as the dressing for a Thai beef salad, although you may want to increase the chilli a little.

Herb dressing

Each herb has its own particular flavour and will work best with a different acid (vinegar or citrus juice) and oil base as suggested below. Sammie says this dressing is great for drizzling around plates—it adds a visual punch. Feel free to experiment, using a combination of lighter herbs—tarragon, chervil, parsley and chives would be delicious with a dash of Dijon mustard and lemon juice. Oregano, rosemary and parsley with a couple of anchovies and lemon juice would be a sublime accompaniment to lamb.

Prep time: 10 minutes
Cooking time: 1 minute

For each dressing use the
    following:

1 cup picked herb leaves
2 tablespoons acid
½ cup oil
pinch of sea salt and freshly
    ground black pepper

Oregano Use lemon juice as your acid and and extra virgin olive oil. Add 1 teaspoon capers, or 3 anchovy fillets.

Parsley Use white wine vinegar as your acid and and extra virgin olive oil

Mint Use red wine vinegar as your acid and extra virgin olive oil. Add a teaspoon of honey

Coriander Use lime juice as your acid and camellia tea oil

Blanch your chosen herb until vibrant green and tender. Drain and refresh in a bowl of iced water. Drain and dry between sheets of absorbent paper
    Place chopped herbs in a blender with all the other ingredients (use only three-quarters of the oil at this stage) and blitz until you have a smooth dressing.

175

Brown rice salad

Edamame beans are immature soybeans still in the pod and are incredibly nutritious. They are popular in Japan and China, where they are often eaten boiled or steamed and salted as a snack. To eat in this way you use your teeth to squeeze the beans from the pod, which is then discarded. You can buy them frozen (either still in their pod or ready-podded) in Asian supermarkets.

Level of effort: 2
Prep time: 20 minutes
Cook time: 45 minutes
Serves 4–6

2 cups brown rice
1 cup edamame beans (frozen)
1 cup peas (frozen or fresh)
1 corn cob
1 red capsicum, roasted, peeled,
    sliced thinly
1 avocado, diced
1 red chilli, sliced thinly
1 cup mizuna leaves

Coriander dressing (p.175)

Put a large saucepan of water on to boil. Wash rice thoroughly. When water is boiling season it with salt and then add the rice. Stir the rice for 1 minute and then leave, at a full boil for at least 30 minutes or until cooked; check every so often to make sure the water hasn't boiled away.

Meanwhile, blanch the beans, peas and corn until they are just tender; drain and set aside. Cut the corn off the cob and mix with the podded beans and peas.

When the rice is cooked, drain thoroughly and tip into a large salad bowl with two times the quantity of the coriander herb dressing. Toss to combine.

Add the bean mixture, capsicum, avocado, chilli and mizuna leaves. Toss gently to combine.

Spiced chickpea salad

You can make this recipe super-quick by using canned chickpeas and simply start at step 2. However, I think the taste of home-cooked chickpeas is worth the extra effort.

Level of effort: 3 (but only a 1 if you use canned chickpeas)
Prep time: 20 minutes (plus overnight soaking)
Cooking time: 1½ hours
Serves 8

1½ cups dried chickpeas, soaked overnight
½ tablespoon olive oil
1 brown onion, sliced thinly
2 cloves garlic, sliced thinly
1 long red chilli, sliced thinly
pinch dried chilli flakes, optional
pinch saffron
½ teaspoon salt
freshly ground black pepper
400g can diced tomatoes
½ cup (125ml) water
½ cup flat leaf parsley leaves, chopped coarsely

Drain chickpeas and rinse thoroughly. Place in a large saucepan of boiling water and simmer 1½ hours or until tender.

Heat the olive oil in a pan and cook onion, garlic and chilli until softened and translucent.

Add dried chilli flakes (adding dried chillies gives a more rounded flavour although you can omit them if you prefer), saffron, salt and pepper and cook for 30 seconds to bring out the flavour of the saffron.

Add drained cooked chickpeas, tomatoes and water and bring to a boil; simmer 20 minutes or until sauce thickens and coats the chickpeas.

Remove from the heat and cool to room temperature. Stir in the parsley just before serving.

Supercharge

Legumes such as chickpeas, lentils, beans and soybeans are among the best plant foods to eat as they can help to reduce our reliance on animal produce. They provide good levels of protein and low GI carbohydrates, and can fulfil either the protein (in a veggie meal) or carb component of a meal. They are packed with nutrients, including soluble fibre, antioxidants, several vitamins and minerals including folate, iron and zinc. The vitamin C in the tomato sauce will help you to absorb these minerals.

Prawn and chicken larb

The herbs used in this recipe are wonderfully fragrant. If you can't find one of them increase the quantities of the ones you have. The flavour will be slightly different, but no less delicious.

Level of effort: 2
Prep time: 15 minutes
Cook time: 15 minutes
Serves 4

2 tablespoons red coral rice
1 tablespoon peanut oil
500g small prawns: half peeled
    and chopped, half left whole
1 stick lemongrass, white part only,
    finely chopped
2 long red chilli, halved and thinly
    sliced
250g chicken mince
½ cup chicken stock
8 green onions, sliced thinly
2 tablespoons lime juice
1 tablespoon fish sauce
⅓ cup coriander leaves
¼ cup mint leaves, torn
¼ cup Thai basil leaves
½ small Chinese cabbage,
    shredded
1 Lebanese cucumber, halved,
    deseeded, sliced
sesame oil, optional

Place the rice in the dry wok and cook over a high heat until lightly toasted. Remove and cool slightly before grinding in a spice grinder or mortar and pestle; set aside.

Heat oil in the same wok. Add whole prawns, lemongrass and chilli and stir-fry for 1 minute or until prawns are just cooked. Remove whole prawns and place on a plate until a little later.

Add chopped prawns and chicken mince and fry until browned. Add stock and onions and simmer for about 5 minutes or until liquid has evaporated. Cool 5 minutes before stirring in the prawns, lime juice, fish sauce and herbs.

Arrange cabbage and cucumber on a platter. Spoon over the mince mixture. Sprinkle over the rice and serve hot or at room temperature with ground dried chilli and sesame oil for guests to add at their discretion.

Red coral rice has been eaten for centuries in Thailand. It's produced by traditional methods that gently polish the grain, so it retains many of the nutrients found in the whole grain, but is tastier and easier to digest. You can also buy it as a fair-trade product. Look for it in the health aisle of the supermarket, whole food stores and good grocers.

Salad niçoise

This delicious salad makes a great lunchbox filler. You can make the dressing and store it in a tiny Tupperware container to add to the salad at the last minute. Pack the whole vegetables and eggs in your lunchbox, and halve them at the last minute to preserve their freshness.

Level of effort 3
Prep time: 30 minutes
Cooking time: 30 minutes
Serves 4

400g kipfler or new potatoes
200g green beans, trimmed
1 clove garlic, unpeeled
4 eggs
2 x 250g tuna steaks
sea salt and freshly ground black
    pepper
1 Lebanese cucumber, deseeded,
    sliced thinly
½ red onion, sliced thinly
⅓ cup black nicoise olives, pitted,
    halved
250g vine-ripened cherry tomatoes
2 tablespoons baby capers, drained
6 anchovy fillets, halved lengthways
½ cup flat-leaf parsley leaves

Dressing
1 tablespoon lemon juice
2 teaspoons red wine vinegar
1 teaspoon Dijon mustard
½ cup (125ml) olive oil
sea salt and freshly ground black
    pepper

Place potatoes in a large saucepan and cover with cold water. Bring to a boil and simmer 12–15 minutes until almost cooked through (test with a skewer). Add beans and garlic to the same pot and boil for the last 4 minutes of the potato cooking time.

Drain potatoes, beans and garlic and rinse under cold running water to refresh. Halve the potatoes, reserve the garlic for the dressing.

Bring a small pot of water to the boil. Once boiling, use a slotted spoon and carefully add the eggs. Boil for 6 minutes. Drain and cool under running water. Peel and set aside.

Preheat a chargrill over a high heat. Brush tuna steaks on both sides with oil and lightly season. Cook on pre-heated chargrill for 2–3 minutes each side or until cooked as desired. Remove from heat, break into large flakes or chunks and set aside.

For the dressing, combine lemon juice, vinegar, garlic and mustard in a medium bowl. Whisk briefly to combine. Place a damp cloth under the bowl and, while whisking, slowly add the olive oil until all is incorporated (emulsified).

To assemble the salad, combine beans, potatoes, cucumber, onion, olives, halved tomatoes, capers, anchovies and parsley in a large bowl. Drizzle a little of the dressing onto four individual serving plates. Arrange a quarter of the salad mixture on each plate and top with tuna and the halved eggs. Drizzle with remaining dressing to serve.

179

CREATE YOUR OWN ... AT THE SANDWICH BAR

As with the salad bar suggestions, these simple steps work at home as well as at the sandwich bar. So when you're out and about or need something fast and tasty at work, you can still make healthy choices.

Step 1: CHOOSE your bread wisely. Look for traditional methods, such as sourdough or flat bread and wholegrain versions where you can. Try sourdough, Mountain bread, wholemeal pita, and wholegrain bread or have an open sandwich on pumpernickel.

I love to have different types of bread but rarely get through the loaf before it's gone stale, particularly when I've bought good-quality bread with no preservatives. The solution? Keep a selection in your freezer. Bread freezes really well and you can then just take out the number of slices you need on a daily basis. Individual slices will defrost in about 10 minutes at room temperature, or cover with a paper towel and microwave for 10–20 seconds.

Step 2: CHOOSE a spread for the bread. Try hummus, mashed avocado, tahini, chutney, mustard, corn relish or even a salsa. Mayo can be fine if you choose a traditional version. If you can find one made with olive oil, so much the better. Better still, make your own! Give store-bought 'light' mayonnaise a miss. If you want to know why, just read the list of ingredients! Similarly, if you're ordering from a sandwich bar skip the mayo—it's hard to know the quality or the ingredients used.

Step 3: ADD your protein-rich food. Try lean meat, chicken or turkey, fish (canned is absolutely fine), egg, cheese (just not everyday) or marinated tofu.

Step 4: PILE on the veggies—green leaves of any sort, sliced beetroot, roasted veggies or antipasto, sliced tomato, capsicum, cucumber, green onions, grated carrot.

Homemade mayonnaise

It's easy to make your own mayonnaise—and this way you'll definitely know what's in it!

Level of effort 2
Prep time: 5 minutes

1 whole egg and 1 egg yolk
1 teaspoon Dijon mustard
1 tablespoon lemon juice
salt and white pepper
100ml extra virgin olive oil
100ml sunflower oil

Place egg and yolk, mustard, juice, salt and pepper in a food processor and process until combined. With the motor operating, gradually add the combined oils in a thin stream until it's all incorporated and the mayonnaise is thick. Check seasoning and add more lemon juice or salt if necessary. This makes about 1 cup of mayonnaise.

Give store-bought 'light' mayonnaise a miss. If you want to know why, just read the list of ingredients!

Hearty barley broth

Level of effort: 1
Prep time: 10 mins
Cooking time: 30 mins

2 teaspoons olive oil
2 cloves garlic, crushed
1 small onion, diced
1 small leek, sliced thinly, leaves
    reserved
½ cup (100g) pearl barley
1 medium carrot, diced
1 stalk celery, diced
1 tablespoon tomato purée
2 cups (500ml) water
2 cups (500ml) stock
1 sprig thyme
1 bay leaf
½ cup coarsely chopped fresh flat-
    leaf parsley
100g diced cooked ham, chicken
    or lamb
½–1 tablespoon lemon juice
sea salt and freshly ground black
    pepper

Heat oil in a large saucepan. Cook garlic, onion, leek and barley for 2 minutes, stirring continuously.

Add carrot, celery and tomato purée and stir for 3 minutes to incorporate all the flavours. Add the water, stock and the thyme, bay and leek leaves tied into a bundle. Bring to a boil, reduce heat and simmer, covered, for about 30 minutes or until barley is tender.

Add parsley, the meat if using, lemon juice and salt and pepper to taste. Cook, stirring continuously, until hot. Serve with baked sourdough croutons.

Curried parsnip soup

Level of effort: 1
Prep time: 10 minutes
Cooking time: 25 minutes

1 tablespoon olive oil
1 onion, chopped
1 green apple, peeled and
    chopped
4 large parsnips, peeled, chopped
1 teaspoon ground coriander
2 teaspoons ground cumin
2 teaspoons garam marsala
1 litre good-quality chicken stock
    (p. 201 or 206)
salt and freshly ground black
    pepper

Heat oil in a large saucepan. Add onion, apple and parsnip and cook for about 5 minutes or until vegetables soften slightly.

Stir in the ground spices and cook until fragrant.

Add stock and simmer about 20 minutes or until vegetables are tender. Cool 10 minutes before puréeing in a blender until very smooth.

Season to taste and serve with snipped chives if desired.

Potato, zucchini, broccoli and feta frittata

Level of effort: 1
Prep time: 20 minutes
Cooking time: 40 minutes
Serves 8 as a snack

2 tablespoons olive oil
600g potatoes, chopped into 1cm
    dice
2 medium brown onions, sliced
    thinly
2 medium zucchini, sliced thinly
150g lightly steamed broccoli
    florets
100g feta cheese, crumbled
¼ cup chopped chives
½ cup flat-leaf parsley leaves,
    sliced thinly
10 free-range or organic eggs
sea salt and freshly ground black
    pepper

Grease and line 22cm deep cake pan. Preheat oven to 160°C.

Sauté potatoes in the oil in a large non-stick pan until browned and starting to soften; transfer to a large bowl using a slotted spoon.

Heat remaining oil in the same pan. Cook onion and zucchini until tender and starting to brown. Transfer to the bowl with the potatoes. Add broccoli, feta, chives, parsley, eggs and salt and pepper and stir well to combine and break up the eggs.

Pour mixture into prepared cake tin; bake in preheated oven for 30 minutes or until frittata is cooked through and golden brown. Cool 5 minutes before serving or cool to room temperature before cutting into bite-sized pieces.

Steak sandwich with caramelised onions and horseradish mayonnaise

There is brown sugar in this recipe and you have my OK to use it! Although too many added refined sugars in our diet are undesirable, adding a little sugar when required to a healthy recipe is absolutely fine. Here it makes all the difference by caramelising the onions making the whole sandwich delicious.

Level of effort: 2
Prep time: 15 minutes
Cooking time: 35 minutes
Serves 4

2 tablespoons olive oil
2 red onions, finely sliced
1 tablespoon dark muscovado
   sugar
sea salt and freshly ground black
   pepper
2 tablespoons balsamic vinegar
2 teaspoons fresh thyme leaves

⅔ cup (200g) real egg mayonnaise
   (preferably olive oil based)
1 tablespoon horseradish
¼ teaspoon dry English mustard

4 minute steaks
8 thin slices sourdough bread,
   toasted
2 vine tomatoes, sliced
butter lettuce

Heat 1½ tablespoons olive oil in a medium saucepan over a medium–low heat. Add onion, cook for 10 minutes or until very soft.

Add the sugar and balsamic vinegar and cook for a further 2–3 minutes until sugar starts to caramelise; add the thyme and season to taste.

Place the mayonnaise in a small bowl, stir in the horseradish and mustard; mix well.

Season steaks liberally with salt and pepper and drizzle with remaining olive oil. Heat a large frying pan until very hot. Add steaks and cook for 2 minutes on each side.

To make the sandwiches, spread some mayonnaise on the cut side of the toasted sourdough bread, followed by steak, onion, tomato and lettuce, finishing with remaining mayonnaise.

185

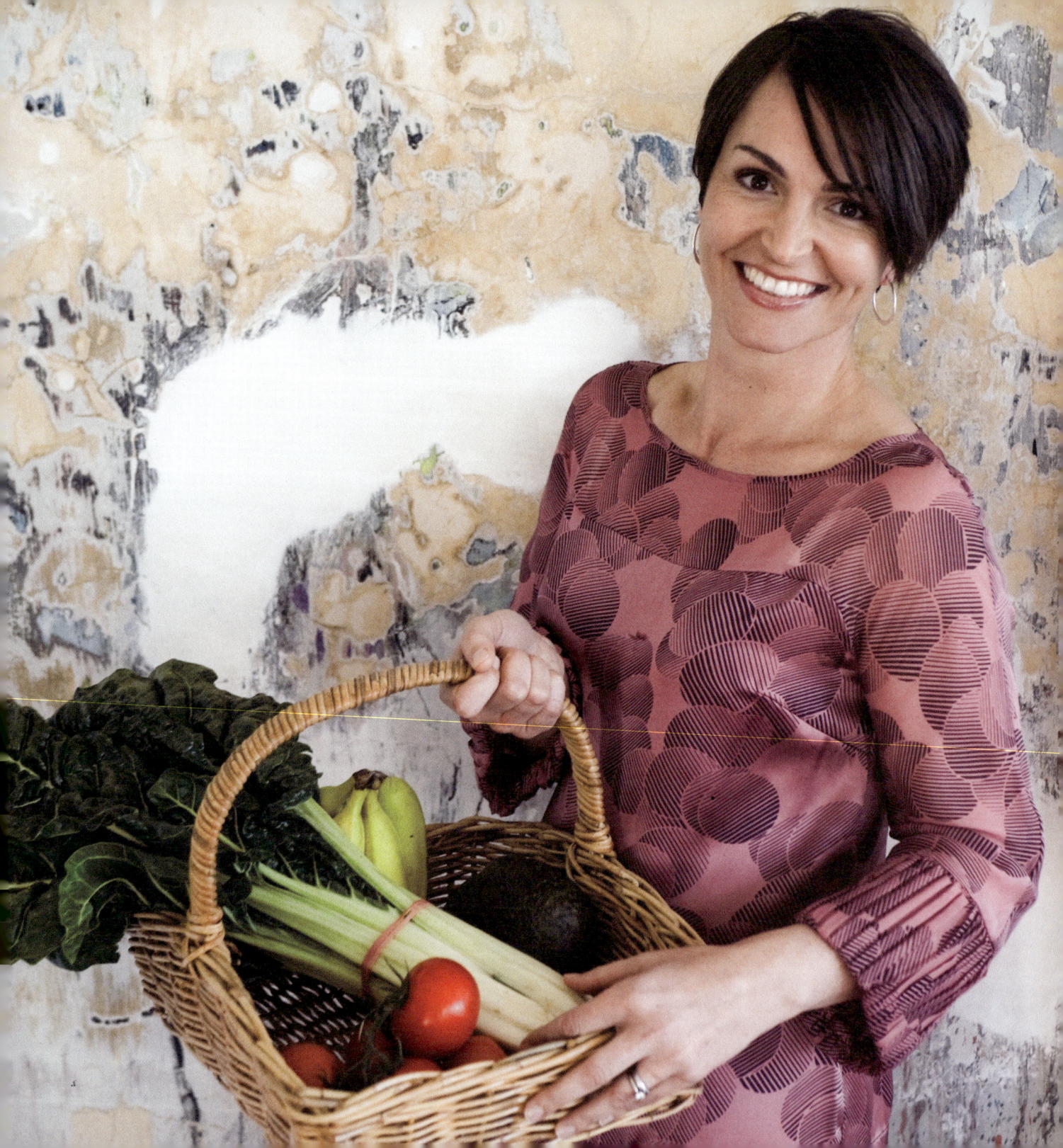

Quinoa, mackerel and spinach kedgeree

This recipe works really well with poached salmon or even canned tuna. To maximise the flavour you can boost the amount of spice—use 2 teaspoons of garam masala and a green chilli.

Level of effort: 2
Prep time: 30 minutes
Cooking time: 35–40 minutes
Serves 4

50g olive oil
2 teaspoons brown mustard seeds
½ teaspoon cumin seeds
1 cinnamon stick
1 large onion (200g) sliced thinly
1½ teaspoons garam masala
½ teaspoon ground turmeric
1½ cups (270g) quinoa
2 cups (500ml) water
1 teaspoon sea salt
freshly ground black pepper
400g smoked mackerel
3 free-range or organic eggs, hard-
    boiled and peeled
100g baby spinach leaves
¼ cup coarsely chopped parsley

Heat oil in large heavy-based frying pan with a lid. Add mustard seeds, cumin and cinnamon and cook 1–2 minutes or until mustard seeds pop.

Add onion and ground spices, cook until onion has softened and started to lightly brown.

Add quinoa, water and salt and pepper. Cover with the lid and boil for 10–15 minutes or until quinoa is tender.

Meanwhile, flake fish into large chunks and cut eggs in half.

Stir fish, spinach and parsley into the quinoa and stir gently until the spinach wilts.

Serve topped with eggs and with some Worcestershire or sweet chilli sauce.

You'll find smoked mackerel in the supermarket fridge, near the smoked salmon.

Supercharge

Smoked and canned fish are a convenient way to boost your omega-3 intake (you should aim to eat oily fish at least twice a week). Smoking fish and meat is one of the oldest methods of food preservation but you won't find the Heart Foundation Tick on these foods because of the large amount of salt used in the smoking process. Despite this, I still recommend using it, in the context of a wholesome natural food diet. If you don't eat many processed foods then your overall salt intake will be within healthy limits despite having smoked fish once a week or so. Read the ingredients list to be sure the product has only fish and salt, and no other additives. Avoid fish (and meat) that has been smoke flavoured with chemicals rather than with traditional methods.

Dinner

Dinner is arguably the most important meal of the day for most of us. It's usually our biggest meal and therefore supplies us with the most nutrients. That also means dinner can throw the whole day out if we get it wrong. The most common mistake is coming home and ravenously devouring the bread bin or cheese box before even the thought of cooking a meal. Make sure that you have enough to eat during the day so that you're not starving when you walk through the door—after a stressful day you might be more likely to pour yourself a glass of chardy and reach for the pizza menu! But cooking can be a great stress reliever. And I promise you whatever the circumstance you will feel infinitely better after a home-cooked, nutrient-charged meal. Feel free to enjoy the glass of chardy while you cook—so long as you can stop at one or two. You also should aim to have at least a couple of alcohol-free nights in your week.

THOROUGHLY MODERN MEAT AND TWO VEG

- Choose a lean cut of meat. An appropriate portion is roughly the size of the palm of your hand. Ideal cuts include kangaroo fillets, beef fillet, lamb backstraps, pork cutlets, veal or chicken (skin and visible fat removed). The beauty of a good-quality cut of meat is that all you need do is season it and either chargrill it to your liking on the stovetop or on the barbie.
- Add some sort of good-quality carbohydrate-rich food. Regular potatoes are fine every now and again, but they do have a high GI. Sweet potatoes are far more nutritious—choose the orange variety for a fabulous beta-carotene hit. Depending on the variety, sweet potatoes have a low GI as well. You could also cook a small serve of pasta, brown rice, freekeh or other wholegrain and flavour simply with some good-quality olive or nut oil, a pinch of sea salt and freshly ground black pepper.
- Finally fill the remaining half of your plate with veggies. In summer you might choose salad dressed with a delicious dressing (see our suggestions on pages 172–5), or in winter simply chop a variety of whatever veggies you have in the fridge or freezer and steam or stir-fry in a good-quality oil. This is a regular meal in our household and I can get it on the table in less than 20 minutes.

FISH FRESH

Follow more or less the same plan for lean meat but use fish instead. The only exception is the more delicate white fish—these tend to be less successful cooked on the grill. I prefer to bake them in the oven, simply flavoured with lemon juice, seasoning and a sprinkle of dried dill or other herbs. Reduce the cooking time by half for the fish and check to see that it is cooked through before removing it from the heat.

CURRY FAVOUR

- Buy a good quality curry paste, add some meat and vegetables and a wholesome, healthy meal can be on the table in half an hour. It takes some cuts of meat longer to cook, but even then the preparation time is minimal. For true curry chefs who like to spend hours preparing spices and making their dishes from scratch (and I like to also, now and again) this may sound sacrilegious but in the name of speed and convenience I give you my permission! Choose a paste that has recognisable ingredients and no artificial colours, flavours or preservatives added. You can always add some fresh ginger or chilli to a bought curry paste to add freshness and pep it up a little. If you do find time to make your own curry pastes, make it in larger batches and freeze in an ice-cube tray—that way you can easily remove 2 or 3 tablespoons when you're in a hurry.
- In a bowl, coat the diced meat with the curry paste. Fry a diced onion in coconut, peanut or camellia tea oil (depending on the flavours of the curry) until softened, add the diced meat and stir until the meat has browned. Then add a can of chopped tomatoes. Simmer on a low heat—20 minutes is enough for chicken while tougher cuts of lamb or beef are best cooked for up to an hour.
- Towards the end of cooking add as many chopped vegetables as you can. Capsicum, cauliflower, okra, peas, green beans, baby corn or corn kernels, carrot, pumpkin, sweet potato and squash all go well in a curry. For added convenience this is one dish where frozen vegetables work well so there is minimal need for fresh ingredients.
- Finally, add either a can of coconut milk or a few spoonfuls of natural yoghurt depending on the curry. Serve with steamed brown rice, basmati rice or Thai red coral jasmine rice.

189

On the table in less than 15 mins...

Rosemary lamb backstraps with chargrilled sweet potato and feta salad

Preheat a barbecue or ridged chargrill pan until very hot.

Brush lamb backstraps with a sprig of rosemary dipped in olive oil and season with salt and pepper. Chargrill for 3 minutes each side so that it is still pink in the middle. Set the lamb aside to rest.

Microwave slices of sweet potato for 3 minutes and brush with the rosemary and oil. Chargrill until browned and tender.

Serve with a salad of baby spinach, slivers of red onion, whole cherry tomatoes and chunks of feta, all dressed with an oregano version of the vinaigrette (p.175).

Poached salmon salad

Bring water to boil in a pan, add a fresh salmon fillet and bring back to the boil. Reduce the heat and simmer for about 4 minutes. Remove the salmon and keep warm.

Throw together a salad of snow pea sprouts, sliced green onions, olives, semi-dried tomatoes, toasted pine nuts, cucumber and sliced red capsicum.

In a jar shake 1 tablespoon of extra virgin olive oil, ½ tablespoon lemon juice, ½ tablespoon pomegranate molasses and a teaspoon of honey. Toss through salad.

Break salmon fillet into chunks and add to the salad. Serve with a slice of wholegrain sourdough bread.

Pomegranate molasses is concentrated pomegranate juice. It comes in a bottle as a dark, thick, sticky liquid with a tart flavour. It's fantastic as a marinade for chicken or pork, or as my favourite to make a tangy salad dressing.

191

Herbed tuna pasta with baby spinach

Cook some penne pasta until al dente.

When the pasta is cooking, heat some olive oil in a pan and add a crushed clove of garlic and finely sliced red onion.

When translucent, add a sliced green capsicum, a handful of sliced mushrooms, a sliced zucchini and sauté for a couple of minutes.

Add a can of cherry tomatoes (or chopped tomatoes), a tablespoon of tomato paste, a splash of white wine and a teaspoon each of dried basil and oregano (if you have fresh herbs to hand, add at the end of cooking to preserve their colour and fragrant aroma). Cook for a few more minutes.

Add a can of tuna and a handful of olives. Toss sauce through the drained pasta, adding a generous handful of baby spinach.

Serve topped with parmesan shavings.

Easy pizza

Preheat the oven to 250°C.

Spread ready-made pizza bases or wholemeal Lebanese or pitta bread with tomato paste, grated good-quality mozzarella, your choice of sliced veggies (try zucchini, capsicum, mushroom, sundried tomato, olives, capers, corn) and crumble over some goat's cheese.

Bake in the oven for 10 minutes, top with rocket leaves and serve.

The supermarket pizza bases usually have preservatives added to increase shelf life. Instead, head to an Italian grocer or deli and buy their own homemade varieties and check the ingredients list for one free of preservatives.

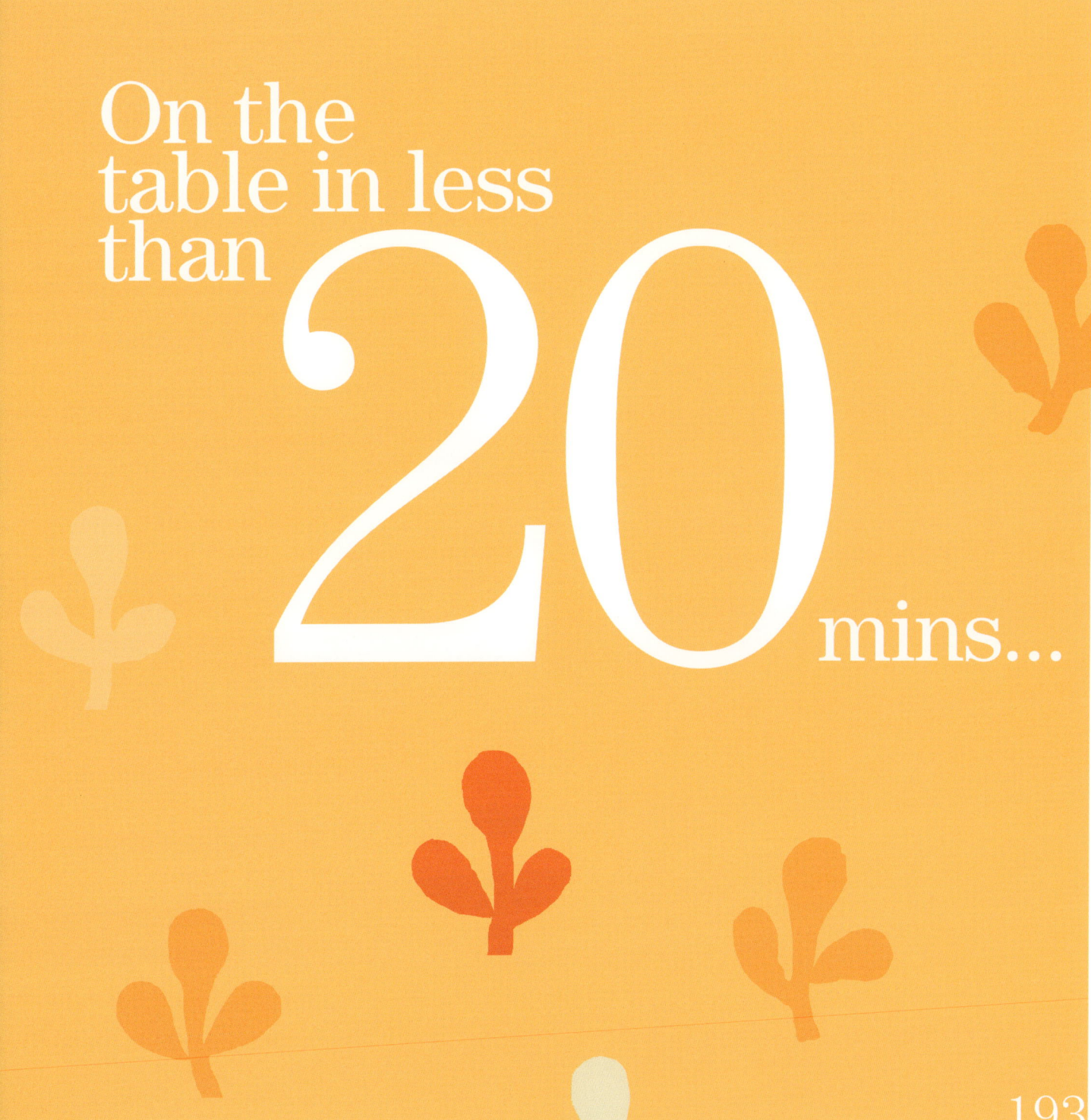

On the
table in less
than

20
mins...

On the table in less than 30 mins...

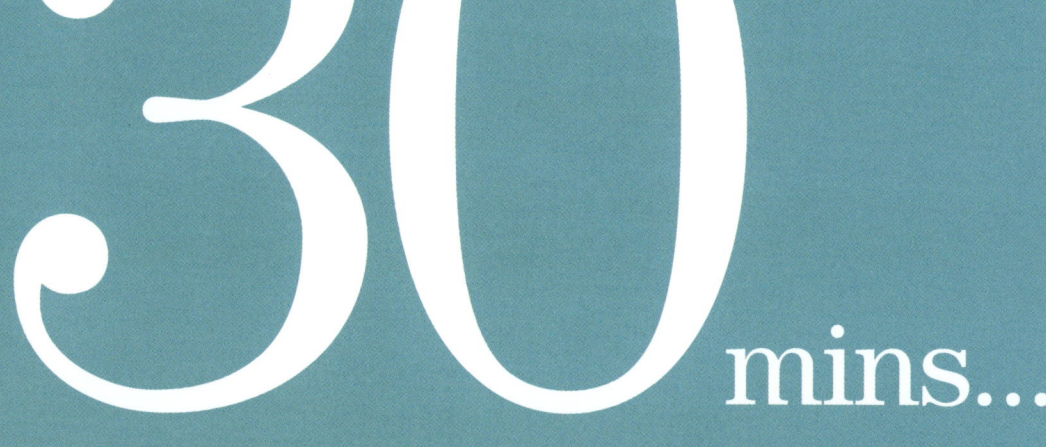

Citrus chicken with tarragon

Preheat oven to 200°C.

Cook some basmati rice.

Take a whole fresh chicken and remove the drumsticks, thighs and wings using a sharp knife by cutting through the joints. Remove the breasts from the bone and cut into two or three parts. Remove the skin from all the chicken pieces. Reserve the carcass and wings for making stock (see p. 201).

Heat some olive oil in an ovenproof casserole dish and brown the chicken pieces.

Remove the chicken to a plate while you sauté a sliced onion and a couple of crushed garlic cloves for a few minutes or until they start to turn translucent.

Add the juice of 1 lemon and ½ an orange, 1 cup of chicken stock and a good pinch of salt. Bring to a boil.

Add the chicken pieces to the stock mixture with 2 sprigs of tarragon and put on the lid.

Bake in the preheated oven for 20 minutes or until chicken is cooked.

Sprinkle with extra chopped tarragon and serve with rice and a green salad.

Kangaroo fajitas

Cut kangaroo fillets (or lean beef or lamb) into strips and mix in bowl with sprinkle of paprika, ground cumin, ground coriander and lemon juice.

Slice an onion and a generous amount of different coloured capsicum into strips.

Heat a little oil and add the kangaroo. Fry for a couple of minutes until just browned and remove from pan.

Add onion and a crushed garlic clove. Once softened add the capsicum and stir-fry for a few minutes.

Add the meat back to the pan along with any juices and a tablespoon or two of tomato paste.

Mash an avocado with a little lemon juice, grate some cheese, wash a few cos lettuce leaves and fill a small jug with natural yoghurt.

Heat a packet of tortilla wraps in the microwave and place all the dishes in the middle of the table for everyone to roll their own fajita wraps.

Take a wrap, spread with avocado, a handful of leaves, a spoonful of the kangaroo veggie mixture, a drizzle of yoghurt and sprinkle of cheese. Fold and eat. Voila! Kangaroo fajitas, Oz-Mex style!

You can buy preservative-free tortillas in good delis.

Broad bean and goat's cheese pasta

Use any green summer vegetables that you fancy—peas, grated zucchini, broccoli, asparagus, rocket, fresh herbs and/or a combination of some or all of them would all work well.

Level of effort 2
Prep time: 15 minutes
Cooking time: 10 minutes
Serves 4

2 cups podded broad beans
2 tablespoons olive oil
1 clove garlic, bruised
5 eschalots, sliced thinly
110g soft goat's cheese
finely grated zest and juice of half
    a lemon
2 tablespoons shredded parsley
freshly ground black pepper
375g whole-wheat spaghetti

Boil broad beans until they are just tender. Drain and rinse under cold water. When they are cool enough to handle, peel off the outer grey layer and discard. Set aside the peeled beans.

Heat half the oil in a saucepan and add the garlic and eschalots. Cook slowly until the eschalots are translucent and the garlic has infused its flavour into the oil. Discard the garlic.

Add two-thirds of the beans to the eschalots with the goat's cheese. Purée or crush with a masher until coarsely crushed. Add the lemon zest, freshly ground black pepper and taste to check the seasoning. Add as much of the lemon juice as you feel necessary—it may only need a teaspoon.

Stir in the remaining beans and the parsley. Set aside.

Boil the pasta in plenty of boiling salted water until al dente. Drain, reserving a little of the cooking water.

Toss the pasta through the broad bean mixture, adding some of the cooking water if necessary to thin the sauce a little. Season with black pepper and serve immediately.

Chickpea and vegetable patties

Level of effort: 3
Prep time: 30 minutes
Cooking time: 15 minutes
Serves 4–6

420g can chickpeas, drained and
    rinsed
2 medium zucchini (240g), coarsely
    grated
1 medium onion (200g), grated
2 medium carrots (240g), coarsely
    grated
1 small sweet potato (250g),
    coarsely grated
1 egg, lightly beaten
1 cup bread crumbs, made from
    sourdough or wholegrain bread
1 clove garlic, crushed
2cm piece ginger, grated
⅓ cup coriander leaves, roughly
    chopped
⅓ cup sesame seeds, toasted
1 teaspoon ground cumin
2 teaspoons ground coriander
salt and pepper
olive oil (for cooking)

In a large bowl roughly mash chickpeas. Add remaining ingredients and mix well. Sit for 10 minutes and mix again (this allows flavours to develop).

Form mixture into 6 large round patties and refrigerate 30 minutes to firm them up (they can be frozen at this stage).

Heat a flat frying pan, brush patties with a little oil and cook on both sides until golden brown.

Serve on sourdough toast topped with tahini, sliced tomato, avocado, rocket and chilli sauce.

Stir-fried Asian greens with marinated tofu

Level of effort 2
Prep time: 10 minutes
Cooking time: 10 minutes
Serves 4

3 garlic cloves, finely sliced
2 large red chillies, seeds removed
    and finely sliced
4cm ginger, finely grated
¼ cup (60ml) soy sauce
2 tablespoons Chinese cooking
    wine or dry sherry

250g block firm tofu, sliced thickly

2 tablespoons peanut oil
6 green onions, cut into 3cm
    lengths
200g snow peas, trimmed and
    sliced lengthways
1 bunch Chinese broccoli, trimmed
    and chopped
1 bunch snake beans, cut into
    2–3cm batons
2 carrots, cut into batons
1½ cups bean sprouts, trimmed
1 tablespoon water
¼ cup Thai basil leaves
¼ cup coriander leaves

Combine garlic, chilli, ginger, soy and cooking wine in a shallow bowl and add the sliced tofu to it to marinade. Set aside at least 1 hour for the flavours to penetrate the tofu.

Heat a wok, add oil and fry onions briefly. Add remaining vegetables and stir-fry until just starting to soften.

In a separate pan, fry the drained tofu (reserving the marinade) until golden brown and slightly crisp. Remove to a plate and keep warm.

Add reserved marinade to the stir-fried vegetables and toss quickly to combine. Bring the mixture to the boil.

Serve with the sliced tofu and steamed doongara or other low-GI rice.

Tomatoes stuffed with pilaf and mushrooms

Use whatever you like to make up the filling of the tomatoes. The rice or quinoa could have been cooked previously (for example, the quinoa pilaf, p. 213), in which case, sauté the vegetables, add the cooked rice or quinoa and just bake the tomatoes in a 220°C oven for only 15 minutes. Vary the vegetables you add according to your own preference. Oregano or rosemary would be delicious herbs to add to the grain mixture.

Prep time: 20 minutes
Cook time: 35 minutes
Serves 6

6 large vine-ripened tomatoes
2 tablespoons camellia tea oil or olive oil
1 medium onion, diced finely
1 large red capsicum, diced finely
½ cup uncooked quinoa (or rice)
400g mushrooms, diced finely
sea salt and freshly ground black pepper
1 teaspoon chopped thyme leaves
100g feta, crumbled
¼ cup chopped flat-leaf parsley
approx 1 cup (250ml) vegetable stock

Preheat oven to 200°C/180°C fan-forced.

Cut the top off each tomato and scoop out the seeds using a teaspoon. Reserve the pulp.

Heat half the oil in a saucepan and cook the onion and capsicum until tender. Add quinoa (or rice) and stir to combine.

In a separate saucepan heat the remaining oil and cook mushrooms until tender. Season well with salt, pepper and thyme.

Divide mushroom mixture among the base of the tomatoes with a little crumbled feta on top.

Add parsley, tomato pulp and pepper to the quinoa (rice) mixture and pack loosely into the tomatoes.

Place the stuffed tomatoes into a snug-fitting baking dish and pour a couple of tablespoons vegetable stock into each tomato. Pour a little extra stock around the base of the tomatoes.

Bake in preheated oven 25 minutes or until tomatoes are tender and the quinoa (or rice) is cooked through. Serve with a crisp green salad.

So many of our culinary skills are being lost as increasing numbers of women spend less time in the kitchen. Previous generations understood economy and knew, for example, how to make the most of every part of a whole chicken. It's sometimes convenient to buy just chicken breasts or thighs, but it's far more cost-effective to buy the whole bird and use it over several meals. In my local supermarket a 500g pack of breast fillets costs only a couple of dollars less than a whole size 16 bird weighing 1.6 kg from the butcher (not to mention the plastics in the extra packaging). Given the rising cost of food, particularly healthy food, we would do well to regain a few of these lost skills.

The recipes that follow make the most of a chicken in several ways. You can poach it to make nutritious stock for a fragrant broth, and meltingly tender meat for a couple of light, delicious meals. Or you can roast it first for intense flavour and then cook up the carcass for more stock. If you don't have time to do it straightaway, you can freeze the carcass and make your stock later. When you have two carcasses you can make a larger batch. Whichever way you go, the results are delectable.

Poached chicken and chicken stock

Prep time: 10 minutes
Cooking time: 50 minutes
Makes approximately 3 litres

1 size 16 chicken
1 teaspoon peppercorns, cracked
  slightly
1 teaspoon salt
2 onions, thickly sliced
3 cloves garlic
4 litres water, approximately

Rinse chicken under running water. Place chicken in a large pot. Cover with the water and slowly bring to a boil.

Skim surface and reduce heat. Add remaining ingredients and simmer for 45 minutes. Remove from heat and cool the chicken in the stock for at least ½ hour.

Carefully remove the chicken and use in the following recipe. Strain the stock through muslin or a clean, damp Chux cloth into a large bowl; reserve for the soup recipe following. Stock can be frozen in 2-cup batches for future use, or refrigerated for 2 days.

White cooked chicken with spring onions and ginger

Level of effort: 1 (if you've already poached
  the chicken)
Prep time: 15 minutes
Cooking time: 5 minutes
Serves 2–4 (with steamed Asian greens)

poached chicken (above)
6 spring onions, chopped finely
4cm piece ginger, finely grated
¼ cup good-quality peanut oil
pinch sea salt

Using a sharp knife, carefully remove the chicken breasts. Remove the skin and slice the chicken about 5mm thick on the diagonal.

Arrange chicken on serving plates. Spoon the combined onions and ginger over the chicken.

Just before you are ready to serve, heat the oil in a small saucepan until smoking. Pour the oil over the onions and ginger to release their wonderful aromas and to remove some of the rawness from the onions.

Serve with steamed Asian greens and rice.

Chicken fresh spring rolls

Level of effort: 3
Prep time: 30 minutes
Cooking time: nil
Makes: 20 rolls

50g bundle of rice vermicelli
¼ cup sweet chilli sauce
juice of 1 lime
1 tablespoon fish sauce
poached chicken, shredded (p. 201)
200g snow peas, trimmed,
    shredded
1 small carrot, peeled, julienne
1 red capsicum, sliced thinly
½ cup coriander leaves
20 rice paper rounds

Place noodles in a large heatproof bowl. Cover with boiling water and stand 10 minutes or until noodles are softened. Drain and then cut them into short lengths using scissors.

Combine sweet chilli, lime juice and fish sauce in the base of a large bowl. Add noodles, chicken, snow peas, carrot, capsicum and coriander and toss to coat in the sauce.

To assemble the rice paper rolls, lay a tea towel on the kitchen bench. Place a roasting tin on the bench behind the tea towel and fill with hot water. Submerge a rice paper round in the hot water for 20–30 seconds (this will vary depending on the heat of the water, but don't make it too hot) until it softens before placing on the tea towel (this will help to absorb excess moisture).

Place about 2 tablespoons of the prepared filling on the bottom third of the rice paper and roll the bottom over it to enclose the filling. Fold the sides in before continuing to roll the rice paper up.

Set aside while you make up the rest of the rice paper rolls.

Serve with extra sweet chilli sauce or a light soy sauce mixed with a little lemon juice.

Light summer broth

Level of effort: 2
Prep time: 15 minutes
Cooking time: 10 minutes

1.5 litres of the chicken stock
3 shallots, finely diced
1 small zucchini, finely diced
⅔ cup peas
60g snow peas, trimmed, sliced
    thinly
½ cup podded broad beans, outer
    grey skin removed
2 tomatoes, peeled, seeded, diced
    finely
1 tablespoon mint leaves, finely
    shredded
juice of half a lemon, or to taste
pinch salt
1 tablespoon tiny basil leaves, to
    garnish

Bring chicken stock to a boil, add shallots and zucchini and boil 2 minutes.

Reduce heat to a gentle simmer and add peas, snow peas and broad beans. Cook 5 minutes or until vegetables are tender.

Add remaining ingredients, the lemon juice and salt to taste, and stir until heated through.

Divide among soup bowls and top with the basil leaves and baked sourdough croutons if desired.

You could add a small handful of tiny pasta (broken spaghetti is fine if you do not have special small pasta shapes) to the soup for a heartier dish. Add pasta to the boiling stock about 3–5 minutes before you add the vegetables.

Chicken roasted with lemon and garlic

Level of effort: 1
Prep time: 10 mins
Cooking time: 1½ hours
Serves 4 (and use the leftovers for the
   beetroot, pumpkin and chicken salad, and
   the carcass for chicken stock, p. 201)

1.8kg chicken
a drizzle of olive oil
6 cloves garlic, unpeeled
1 lemon
I small bunch thyme
2 teaspoons sea salt flakes
cracked black pepper

Preheat the oven to hot (220°C/200°C fan-forced).
Wash the chicken under cold water and pat dry with absorbent paper.

Season the chicken inside the cavity liberally with salt and pepper. Bruise the cloves of garlic and cut the lemon into wedges.

Stuff the garlic, half of the lemon and the thyme inside the chicken. Squeeze the remaining lemon juice over the chicken, sprinkle with salt and pepper and drizzle with olive oil. Place the chicken, breast-side down, on a rack in an oiled heavy-based baking dish. Roast in the preheated oven for 30 minutes.

Turn the chicken over and roast a further 50 minutes. Test to see if it is cooked through by piercing the thigh with a skewer. The juices should run clear.

Once chicken is cooked through, remove from oven, cover and rest for 10 minutes to allow the juices to settle back into the meat and for the muscle fibres to relax (this makes for more tender meat).

Beetroot, pumpkin and chicken salad with parsley and walnut dressing

Level of effort: 2
Prep time: 20 minutes
Cooking time: 1 hour

8 small beetroot, trimmed
700g butternut pumpkin, peeled, cut into large chunks
1 tablespoon olive oil
sea salt and freshly ground black pepper
pinch dried chilli flakes, optional
150g baby spinach
400g (approx. 2 cups) cooked chicken, left over from the roast, roughly shredded or chopped
100g feta, crumbled
¾ cup (75g) toasted walnuts

Parsley and walnut dressing
2 tablespoons light olive oil
2 tablespoons walnut oil
2 tablespoons finely chopped parsley
¼ cup (60ml) lemon juice
1 teaspoon wholegrain mustard
1 small clove garlic, crushed, optional

Preheat oven to moderately hot.

Place beetroot in a small shallow baking dish. Roast uncovered for 15 minutes.

Combine pumpkin and oil, salt, pepper and chilli flakes, if using, and roast on a separate baking dish for a further 40 minutes until vegetables are tender.

Using gloves, peel beetroot while still warm. Halve or quarter depending on their size. Combine in a large bowl with all dressing ingredients.

Arrange pumpkin, spinach, chicken, feta and walnuts on a large platter. Spoon the beetroot and dressing over the top.

205

Roast chicken stock

Level of effort: 1
Prep time: 5 minutes
Cooking time: 1½ hours
Makes approx. 2 litres

carcass from roast chicken
2 medium carrots, chopped
    coarsely
1 brown onion, skin on, halved
½ bulb of garlic, halved
1 stick celery, chopped coarsely
½ teaspoon black peppercorns
2 stalks parsley
2 bay leaves
pinch salt
water

Place all the ingredients (except the water) into a large saucepan. Add enough water to cover the ingredients by about 1cm. Bring to a boil, reduce heat and simmer for 1½ hours.

Remove the stock from the heat and cool at least 30 minutes before straining through a fine sieve. Refrigerate or freeze until required.

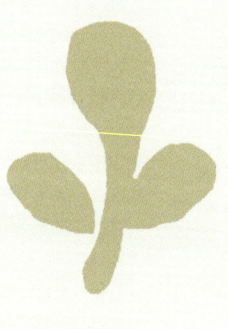

Wild mushroom, leek and barley risotto

Level of effort: 2
Prep time: 20 minutes
Cooking time: 25 minutes
Serves 4–6

20g dried porcini mushrooms,
    soaked in boiling water for 15
    minutes
1.3 litres chicken stock from roast
    chicken
1½ tablespoons olive oil
2 leeks, finely sliced
3 cloves of garlic, peeled and finely
    chopped
1 tablespoon thyme
2 cups (400g) barley, soaked in 2
    cups water for 30 minutes
1 glass of dry white wine
1 tablespoon olive oil, extra
150g shimeji mushrooms
150g Swiss brown mushrooms,
    sliced thickly
freshly ground black pepper
100g goat's cheese
2 tablespoons freshly grated
    Parmesan cheese
¼ cup chopped parsley

Soak the mushrooms and put stock on to heat.

In a separate large heavy based saucepan, heat the oil. Add the leek and garlic and cook, stirring until translucent. Add drained barley and stir to coat it in the vegetable juices.

Add the wine; let it bubble and be absorbed by the barley. Add a ladleful of the hot stock and stir over a gentle heat until the barley absorbs it. Continue to add the stock, a ladleful at a time, until the barley is cooked (you may need to add a little more stock or hot water). Remove from the heat and cover to keep warm.

Drain the porcini mushrooms, saving their soaking liquid and chop coarsely. Fry garlic and thyme with the Swiss browns and shimeji mushrooms in a non-stick frying pan until they are golden.

Stir the drained porcini liquid and remaining stock into the risotto with the cheeses and stand one minute for the flavours to combine.

Stir in the mushrooms and herbs and serve immediately.

207

Grilled chicken with braised peas, broad beans and lettuce

Prep time: 15 minutes
Cooking time: 20 minutes
Serves 4

4 small chicken breasts
salt and pepper
juice of half a lemon
1 tablespoon olive oil

2 teaspoons olive oil
1 bunch green onions (spring
    onions, shallots), thinly sliced
3 cloves garlic, crushed
½ cup (125ml) dry white wine
½ cup (185ml) chicken stock
1 cos lettuce, tough outer leaves
    removed (or used in a salad),
    shredded finely
1 cup peas
1 cup podded broad beans
    (approximately 400g unpodded
    weight)
salt and pepper
2 tablespoons mint, chopped finely

Season chicken with salt and pepper, lemon juice and a drizzle of olive oil.

Heat a chargrill pan and cook chicken for 4 minutes each side or until golden brown and just cooked through. Transfer to a warm plate, cover, and rest while you cook the braised vegetables.

Heat the 2 teaspoons of olive oil and add the onions and garlic, cooking until translucent.

Add wine and bring to a boil, simmering until wine has evaporated. Add lettuce, peas and broad beans and stir to coat in the juices.

Add hot chicken stock and cover pot with lid. Simmer for 5–10 minutes or until peas and beans are just cooked. Stir in the mint.

To serve, slice chicken thickly and serve on top of braised vegetables.

Freekeh tabouleh with za'tar grilled chicken breast

This recipe works just as well with lamb or fish. Za'tar is a Middle Eastern spice blend of toasted sesame seeds, sumac, thyme and a little salt with a magical flavour. It is widely available in Middle Eastern grocers and some delis and supermarkets. You can also add a finely chopped Lebanese cucumber to the tabouleh for an extra-fresh flavour.

Level of effort: 2
Prep time: 30 minutes
Cooking time: 10 minutes
Serves 4

4 small chicken breasts
¼ cup za'tar
juice of half a lemon
olive oil

¼ cup freekeh
juice of 2 lemons
½ cup olive oil
sea salt and freshly ground black
    pepper
large pinch of cumin, optional
2–3 bunches Italian parsley, picked
    and finely chopped (6 cups
    chopped)
5 medium vine-ripened tomatoes,
    finely chopped
3 spring onions, finely chopped
small bunch mint, finely chopped

Combine chicken and za'tar in a large bowl with the lemon juice and 2 teaspoons of olive oil. Set aside while you make the tabouleh.

Boil freekeh for about 15 minutes or until tender. Meanwhile, combine lemon juice, oil, salt and pepper in a large bowl and add cumin, if using.

Drain the cooked freekeh and add it to the dressing while still warm (it will absorb some of the flavours).

When ready to serve, preheat a chargrill pan to very hot. Cook the chicken 4 minutes each side or until cooked as desired. Set aside to rest in a warm place.

Add parsley, tomato, spring onion and mint to the freekeh and toss to combine, adjusting the seasoning to taste.

Slice the chicken thickly and serve with a generous helping of the tabouleh.

Lamb and apricot tagine

Level of effort: 2
Prep time: 25 minutes
Cooking time: 1 hour 50 minutes
Serves 4–6

1 tablespoon olive oil
4 French-trimmed lamb shanks
1 large onion (250g), chopped
3 cloves garlic, sliced thinly
3cm piece ginger, peeled, finely
    grated
2 teaspoons ground coriander
¼ teaspoon turmeric
400g can chopped tomatoes
½ cup (125ml) water
1 tablespoon honey
1 cinnamon stick
1 teaspoon salt
½ cup (70g) organic dried apricots
2 tablespoons lemon juice
300g peeled pumpkin, chopped
    into 2cm pieces
¼ cup (35g) blanched almonds
⅓ cup coriander sprigs

Preheat oven to 180°C (160°C fan-forced).

Heat oil in a large pan. Add lamb shanks, cook until well browned all over.

Transfer lamb shanks to a tagine or ovenproof dish.

Add onions, garlic and ginger to the same pan, cooking until softened and translucent. Add coriander, turmeric, tomatoes, water, honey, cinnamon, salt and apricots. Bring to the boil, then pour mixture over lamb shanks in dish.

Cover the dish, transfer to the oven and cook for 1 hour.

Remove lamb from oven. Add lemon juice and pumpkin and cover. Return to oven for another 30 minutes.

Remove lid, add almonds and cook for a further 15 minutes or until lamb is very tender.

Scatter with coriander and serve with steamed freekeh, couscous or mashed sweet potatoes.

Lemon, anchovy and garlic roasted lamb

Level of effort: 2
Prep time: 15 minutes
Cooking time: 1¾ hours
Serves 6 with leftovers, 8 without

2 kg leg of lamb
2 garlic cloves, sliced thinly
2 sprigs rosemary, leaves picked off
8 anchovy fillets
2 lemons, juiced
1 teaspoon sea salt
freshly ground black pepper
½ cup (125ml) dry white wine
½ cup (125ml) water
1–2 teaspoons redcurrant jelly, optional
¼ cup chopped flat-leaf parsley

Preheat oven to 240°C (220°C fan-forced).

Trim any excess fat from lamb and pierce all over with the tip of a sharp knife to make small holes. Push sliced garlic, chopped rosemary leaves and pieces of anchovy into each of the holes.

Rub the lemon juice, salt and pepper all over the lamb and place on a rack in a roasting pan. Add ½ cup white wine and ½ cup water and roast in preheated oven 30 minutes. Reduce heat to 200°C (180°C fan-forced) and roast a further 1¼ hours or until lamb is cooked as desired. Remove from oven and cover lightly with foil to rest for 15–20 minutes to allow juices to settle back into the meat.

Pour juices into a small saucepan and bring to a boil. Add a small teaspoon of redcurrant jelly if desired, and stir in the parsley. Serve over the carved lamb.

 **Any leftover lamb can be removed from the bone and used in the lamb tagine, or instead of beef in the beef dopiaza recipe overleaf. Just omit the meat-browning stage and the dish will only take 30 minutes to cook.**

Beef dopiaza

Level of effort: 2
Prep time: 15 minutes
Cook time: 2 ½ hours
Serves 6

4 large brown onions, peeled
olive oil
1.2kg skirt steak, diced into 3cm
    cubes
1 cinnamon stick
1 teaspoon cardamom pods
½ teaspoon ground cloves
2 teaspoons cumin seeds, crushed
1 tablespoon coriander seeds,
    crushed
1 teaspoon fenugreek seeds
½ teaspoon ground turmeric
5 garlic cloves, crushed
6cm piece ginger, grated
½ cup plain yoghurt
2 cups (500ml) water
2 long green chillies, chopped
    finely, or ½ teaspoon cayenne
1 teaspoon sea salt
½ teaspoon garam masala

Thinly slice three of the onions and cook in 2 teaspoons of oil and 2 tablespoons water until very tender and browned. Remove from pan and set aside.

Dice remaining onion; set aside.

Add beef in batches and cook until browned all over. Remove beef from pan and add to the onions.

Add oil and the spices, diced onion, garlic and ginger and cook until onion softens and the spices are fragrant.

Reduce heat to medium, add yoghurt a spoonful at a time, stirring to combine.

Once all the yoghurt is added, return meat and onions to the pan with any of their juices, the water, the chopped chillies (or cayenne) and the salt.

Stir to combine and bring to a gentle simmer. Partially cover and simmer until beef is tender (1½ to 2 hours).

Add the garam masala and check seasoning. Serve with quinoa pilaf.

Quinoa pilaf

Level of effort: 1
Prep time: 5 minutes
Cook time: 20 minutes
Serves 6

1 teaspoon olive oil
1 small onion, sliced thinly
1 clove garlic, bruised
3 cardamom pods
1½ cups quinoa
2 cups (500ml) chicken stock

Heat olive oil in a medium saucepan and cook onion and garlic until onion is just translucent.

Add cardamom pods and quinoa and cook, stirring to coat the quinoa in the oil and juices.

Add stock, cover and bring to a boil. Once the stock is boiling, reduce heat to a gentle simmer and cook 15 minutes or until the stock has been absorbed and the quinoa is tender. Serve with Beef Dopiaza.

Kangaroo bolognese sauce

I'm a huge fan of kangaroo meat. It's exceptionally lean, so take care not to let it dry out. The addition of the milk or stock will help. You could also cook this sauce in a slow cooker over the course of the day, or cover it with a round of baking paper (a cartouche) and bake it covered in a low (120°C) oven for 3 hours.

Level of effort: 2
Prep time: 20 minutes .
Cooking time: 2 hours
Serves 8

1½ tablespoons olive oil
1 large onion, finely diced
1 clove garlic, crushed
2 sticks celery, finely diced
800g kangaroo mince
Salt and pepper
1–2 tablespoons tomato paste
¾ cup (185ml) red wine
2 x 400g cans diced tomatoes
1 cup (250ml) chicken stock or
    milk

Heat oil in a large saucepan. Add onion, garlic, celery and carrot and cook until vegetables soften and are translucent.

Add mince and cook, stirring until it browns and breaks up a little. Add tomato paste, stir well and cook 1 minute. Add wine and simmer until reduced by half.

Add tomatoes and stock. Bring to a boil. Reduce heat to a gentle simmer and leave to cook, partially covered, for 1½ hours or until sauce is reduced and thick. Check seasoning.

 **This sauce can be made in advance and frozen or refrigerated until required. It's also a good sauce to freeze in batches. This quantity should feed eight as sauce for pasta.**

214

Warm lentil and roasted vegetable salad with kangaroo or goat's cheese croutons

Level of effort: 2
Prep time: 15 minutes
Cooking time: 20 minutes
Serves 6

1½ cups (300g) puy lentils, or
    Australian blue lentils
1 red capsicum
2 medium zucchini, sliced thinly
2 tablespoons olive or avocado oil
finely grated zest and juice of 1
    lemon
1 tablespoon finely chopped fresh
    thyme, extra
sea salt and freshly ground black
    pepper
100g baby rocket leaves

For kangaroo option:
6 kangaroo fillets (approximately
    150g meat per person)
2 tablespoons balsamic vinegar
1 tablespoon finely chopped fresh
    thyme
2 cloves garlic, crushed

For goat's cheese croutons
    option:
6 small slices sourdough bread
200g soft fresh goat's cheese

Cook lentils in a large saucepan of boiling water for about 15 minutes or until tender.

While lentils are cooking, preheat a chargrill pan and cook lightly oiled capsicum and zucchini until tender. Remove to a plate and cover to keep warm. After about 5 minutes the skin of the capsicum should peel away easily. Slice the capsicum thinly.

Combine oil, lemon zest and juice, thyme and salt and pepper in a large salad bowl.

Drain lentils and rinse under hot water. Toss the lentils into the dressing and toss well to combine. Gently fold in the capsicum, zucchini and rocket. Top the salad with either the kangaroo or the goat's cheese croutons.

FOR KANGAROO
Combine kangaroo, vinegar, thyme and garlic in large bowl. Cover and marinate for 15 minutes.

Chargrill the kangaroo on the heated grill plate for 2 minutes each side, taking care not to overcook or it will become tough.

Transfer to a warm plate and rest the meat 5 minutes. Slice thickly on an angle.

FOR GOAT'S CHEESE CROUTONS
Chargrill the slices of sourdough for 1 minute each side or until golden and crisp.

Spread goat's cheese over one side of the toasted bread. If desired, place goat's cheese toasts under a grill so that the cheese slightly melts.

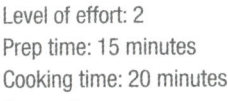 **The lentil salad can be made in advance and served cold if you prefer. The dish can be transformed into a stunning vegetarian meal with minimum fuss by omitting the kangaroo and serving it with the goat's cheese croutons.**

215

Soba noodles and chargrilled salmon with edamame and wakame

Level of effort: 2
Prep time: 10 minutes
Cooking time: 15 minutes
Serves 4

2 cups (500ml) chicken stock
¼ cup (60ml) mirin
2 tablespoons tamari
½ teaspoon sesame oil

300g packet soba noodles
1 cup podded edamame beans
2 bok choy, shredded (stalk and
    leaves kept separate)
2 tablespoons dried wakame
3 green onions, thinly sliced on an
    angle
2 tablespoons sesame seeds,
    lightly toasted

2 teaspoons camellia tea oil
4 x 150g salmon fillets

Combine stock, mirin, tamari and sesame oil in a saucepan. Heat gently and check for seasoning. It may need a little more of one of the ingredients, or a dash of lime juice, depending on personal taste.

Meanwhile, bring a large pot of salted water to a boil. Add soba noodles and cook until al dente; drain and rinse under cold running water. Drain again.

Blanch the edamame beans and bok choy stalks until tender and remove from the water using a slotted spoon. Blanch the bok choy leaves until just tender; drain.

Rehydrate the wakame (seaweed) in a bowl of warm water for 10 minutes; drain.

Heat oil in large non-stick frying pan and cook salmon, skin-side down 4 minutes. Turn and cook a further 3 minutes or until cooked as desired. Remove fish from the pan.

Arrange the noodles in the centre of four bowls. Arrange the blanched vegetables and green onions around the edge of the bowl. Place the salmon, skin-side up, on the noodles and sprinkle with toasted sesame seeds.

Turning Japanese

These wonderful ingredients are not as exotic as you might think. They can be found variously in the Asian foods aisle in your supermarket, in Asian grocers and health food stores.

Mirin is a low alcohol, sweetened rice wine with a delicate flavour used extensively in Japanese cuisine.

Soba noodles are made from buckwheat flour. This is gluten free, yet many soba noodles have wheat flour added. If you're on a gluten-free diet then read the ingredients list. Soba noodles are a delicious low GI choice.

Tamari is a Japanese version of soy sauce, the major difference being it contains no wheat. Look for one that is naturally brewed and not the cheap versions that are artificially flavoured and coloured.

Wakame is a popular type of seaweed with a mild taste. Seaweed can be incredibly nutritious and is one of few foods to provide iodine, that overlooked nutrient often lacking in women's diets.

Whole baked fish with Moroccan roasted vegetables

Level of effort: 3
Prep time: 30 minutes
Cooking time: 1 hour
Serves 6

2–3 tablespoons olive oil
1 large brown onion, sliced thinly
3 large vine-ripened tomatoes,
    chopped coarsely
2 red capsicums, cut into 3cm
    strips
½ teaspoon dried chilli flakes, to
    taste
1½ teaspoons cumin seeds, to
    taste
½ preserved lemon, rinsed,
    chopped
½ cup kalamata olives
Sea salt and black pepper
1 cup flat-leaf parsley leaves
½ cup coriander leaves
1 x 2 kg red emperor or snapper,
    scaled and gutted, fins trimmed

Preheat oven to 240°C (220°C fan-forced).

Combine oil, onion, tomatoes, capsicum, chilli flakes and cumin in a bowl. Remove one third to a baking tray. Bake in pre-heated oven 20 minutes or until just tender. Remove from oven and tip into a bowl. Cover with plastic wrap.

Reduce oven temperature to 200°C (180°C fan-forced).

Combine remaining vegetables with, lemon, olives, salt, pepper and half of the herbs in a large bowl. Tip into a large roasting tray lined with baking paper. (Must be large enough to hold the snapper.)

Cut three deep diagonal slashes into each side of the fish, and then repeat in the opposite direction to create a diamond pattern on each side of the fish.

Lay fish on top of the vegetables. Cover tightly with baking paper and foil.

Cook fish and vegetables in preheated oven 30 minutes. Remove foil and continue to cook a further 30 minutes until the eye is opaque and the flesh is flaking and coming away from the bone when pressed with a knife.

Meanwhile, remove skins from pre-baked vegetables and purée with an extra teaspoon of dried chilli flakes and 1 tablespoon of lemon juice to make the harissa paste. Season to taste and set aside.

When fish is cooked, carefully lift it out of the baking tray and onto a platter. Cover to keep warm.

Increase oven temperature to 240°C (220°C fan-forced). Return the vegetables to the oven and allow them to brown. Toss the parsley into the vegetables and serve them with the fish and harissa.

 Herby couscous or freekeh would be a delicious carb choice to complete this meal.

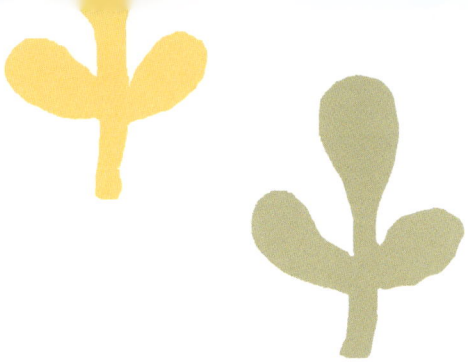

Mussels with tomatoes and rosemary

This recipe is written to cook in two batches because it can be hard to find a saucepan big enough to hold the mussels comfortably in order that they cook properly. You can cook them at the same time if you have two large saucepans that can comfortably contain half the mussels each, or use large wok with a lid.

Level of effort: 2
Prep time: 20–30 minutes
Cooking time: 8–10 minutes
Serves 6

1.5 kg small black mussels
2 tablespoons olive oil
1 medium brown onion, sliced
    thinly
2 cloves garlic, roughly chopped
1 cup (250ml) dry white wine
2 sprigs rosemary
4 ripe roma tomatoes, deseeded
    and diced
salt and black pepper
½ bunch chives, coarsely chopped
¼ cup flat-leaf parsley leaves,
    coarsely chopped

Scrub mussels and remove beards. Set aside.

Heat a large saucepan until very hot. Add half the oil, onion and garlic and cook 1–2 minutes until softened and lightly coloured.

Add half the mussels, wine and rosemary. Cover and cook 5–8 minutes over high heat or until all mussels have opened.

Remove mussels to a large warmed serving bowl with a slotted spoon. Cover to keep warm.

Repeat process with remaining onion, garlic, wine, rosemary and mussels. Add to the mussels already cooked.

Combine juices from both batches and place over a high heat. Add tomatoes, a little salt and plenty of freshly ground black pepper and the herbs. Bring back to a boil and immediately pour over the mussels. Serve with crusty sourdough or rye bread.

Supercharge

We would all do well to eat more mussels. They're a sustainable seafood source (in most areas of Australia you can buy local ones, so food miles are not an issue) and nutritionally they are a perfect source of protein and rich in iron, zinc and iodine, frequently lacking in a woman's diet. They're also cheap compared with meat and fish and they cook really quickly. This recipe is even quicker if you buy the sealed bags of ready-washed and bearded mussels—they're great value for less than $10 for 1 kg.

Sweet treats

Most of us love something sweet – and by choosing sweet treats with the best quality ingredients, you can be sure they enhance your healthy diet. This means no low-fat or diet desserts from the supermarket, or pre-packaged mixes full of additives and refined ingredients. Besides, it's far more economical to make desserts yourself.

These recipe suggestions are both mouth-watering and nutritious. With ingredients such as fresh fruit and dark chocolate, what a delicious way to achieve an antioxidant boost!

FRUIT AND YOGHURT COMBOS

This is the sweet treat I enjoy most often. Commercial fruit yoghurts are generally full of ingredients I don't want to eat, and I've yet to find one that has no sugar or artificial sweetener added. So I make my own. I love to use sheep's milk yoghurt – the thick creamy taste is perfect with fruit. Yes, it contains some fat but it's a natural, minimally processed food and in the context of a healthy, wholesome diet it wins my vote.

Here are my favourite combos:

1 Simply chop whatever fruit you have and serve topped with a generous dollop of natural yoghurt.

2 Puree in the blender a box of frozen berries and mix through natural yoghurt. Sweeten tarter berries with a little honey or maple syrup.

3 Poach a mixture of sliced apples, pears and any combination of dried fruit including dried plums (prunes) and apricots, in a little water. I do this in a low oven for about an hour, or in the slow cooker over 6 hours. The mixture will then keep in the fridge for several days. Top with the yoghurt for a sweet treat, a dessert or a quick brekkie.

DARK CHOCOLATE STRAWBERRIES

These are so simple and inexpensive to make. Just melt a block of dark chocolate (70% cocoa or higher) in a bowl over a pan of just-boiling water. Turn off the heat as soon as the chocolate is melted or you risk burning it. Then simply dip your strawberries into the melted chocolate and lay on a tray lined with baking paper. (100g block of chocolate will coat roughly 10 strawberries.) Pop the tray into the fridge to set the chocolate. They'll keep in the fridge for a few days so they're perfect to make before a dinner party for a quick, delicious and pretty healthy dessert.

HOT COCOA

Drinking chocolate powder is the usual ingredient for a hot chocolate, but most contain added sugar and often flavourings, colourings and other undesirable additives. Instead buy pure unadulterated cocoa powder. This is more like the real thing that the Mayans reportedly drank thousands of years ago and it contains all of the antioxidants and none of the saturated fat or sugar found in most modern chocolate products.

Put 1-2 teaspoons of cocoa powder into a mug and pour over a little boiling water. Mix into a paste before adding hot low fat milk to fill and stir well. I like the slightly bitter chocolately taste, but if you prefer you can add a teaspoon of honey to sweeten.

Orange and almond semolina cake

I've borrowed this recipe from my friend and colleague the Food Coach Judy Davie because I love it so much and it's pretty much the healthiest cake I've encountered. It uses semolina and almond meal in place of white flour, which are both more nutritious and have a lower GI, and uses honey in place of refined sugar. It's sensational as a dessert served with orange segments, a dollop of thick natural yoghurt and a drizzle of pure maple syrup.

Level of effort: 3
Prep time: 30 mins
Cooking time: 1½ hours (plus 1 hour
    cooking time of oranges)
Serves 10

3 oranges
¾ cup semolina
1½ cups ground almond meal
1 tablespoon low allergy baking
    powder
6 egg whites
3 egg yolks
½ cup honey
blanched almond halves

Place the whole oranges in a pan and cover with water. Bring to the boil, reduce to simmer and cook for 1 hour.

When the oranges are cool enough to handle, remove the skin and pith from one orange and place in a food processor with the other two whole oranges.

Preheat the oven to 180°C.

Combine the semolina, almond meal and baking powder together in a bowl. Beat the egg whites until stiff and set aside.

In a separate bowl, beat the egg yolks into the honey.

Beat the almond meal and semolina in with the egg yolk mix and quickly add the orange puree. Fold the egg whites through the cake mixture.

Pour into a small lined cake tin and place blanched almonds over the top to decorate. Cook at 180°C for the first 15 minutes, then reduce the temperature to 150°C and cook for a further 75 minutes.

Leave to cool in the tin for 5 minutes before turning out onto a wire rack. It's delicious served while still warm or over the next couple of days at room temperature.

Chocolate fruit fondue

There are not many times you will find cream in my fridge, but this recipe is worth the extravagance. Cream is indeed high in saturated fat and not something I recommend you eat regularly, but on the other hand it's wholly natural, with no chemical additives and infinitely preferable to a factory-made, low fat, additive-laden diet alternative. The point is don't eat it often but have the real thing when you do.

You need to add the cream to the chocolate to keep the right consistency of the fondue; without it you'll end up with a thick lumpy mess. This is a perfect dessert for a dinner party – the lightness of the fruit is matched by the richness of the chocolate fondue. You won't need much to feel indulged.

Level of effort: 1
Prep time: 15 mins
Cooking time: 10 mins

Your choice of fruit, e.g. whole
    strawberries, chunks of
    pineapple, slices of pear or
    apple, chunks of banana,
    sections of orange or pink
    grapefruit.
300g best quality dark chocolate
    (minimum 70% cocoa)
150ml pure cream
2 tablespoons liquor of your choice
    (optional)

Prepare the fruit into bite size chunks and place on platter.
Heat the cream to near boiling in a pan on the stovetop.
    Break the chocolate into pieces and place in the fondue pot over a low heat. Pour over the hot cream. Add the liquor if using and stir well to melt chocolate and combine.
    Serve immediately with fondue forks for easy dipping.

223

Here are the best options on those nights where

Take
it
away

you order ... *takeaway!*

Asian stir-fries These basically consist of meat, chicken or seafood and veggies cooked quickly with different types of sauces. The rice is the downfall here, being very high GI and a poor source of nutrients other than carbohydrates. Try to have only a small serve or skip it altogether. Or you can cook your own brown rice at home while you wait for the delivery. There are a few delivery menus that include brown rice – this may not be low GI but is a more nutritious option none the less.

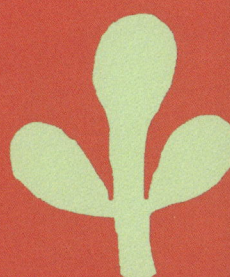

Asian noodles Stir-fried noodles with your choice of meat, chicken, seafood and veggies with sauce. I always ask for extra veggies. Noodles, like pasta, have a low GI so this is a good filling option.

Barbecue chicken Serve with either a large salad (Greek, tabouleh, green) or a tub of roast veggies. If you have veggies in the fridge, then just pick up the chicken from the shop, remove the skin, and throw together your own homemade salad. Skip the chips too! Fill up on extra veggies or salad instead.

Sushi Although sushi is made with white rice it still has a low GI. The combination of fish, seafood and seaweed also provides precious iodine and omega-3 fats.

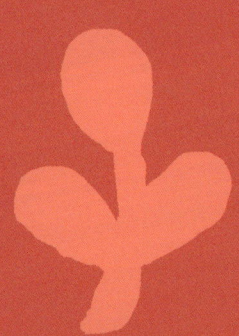

Real Italian pizza By that I'm talking about the thin crispy base with a little cheese and lots of veggies on top. Serve with a large side salad including plenty of green leaves such as rocket and/or spinach, and any other veggies. This is a totally different meal from the pizza-chain monstrosities with stuffed cheese crusts, mountains of fatty meat toppings and buckets of soft drink accompaniments.

Grilled fish Most fish and chip shops offer deep-fried or grilled fish. Go for grilled, add a large salad, or you could quickly stir-fry bok choy or barbecued corn (offered at many good fish shops). It's a fabulously healthy and fast takeaway meal.

Now you know the essential steps towards inner health and outer beauty, go ahead and use them! Strike while the iron is hot. You can be the woman who feels energised, looks her fabulous best, jumps at the chance to move and takes enormous pleasure from eating well. You can take control of your life and work towards a healthier, happier and more vital you. Who knows what you can achieve? Good luck on your journey.

Let me know how you go by visiting me at:
www.joannamcmillanprice.com

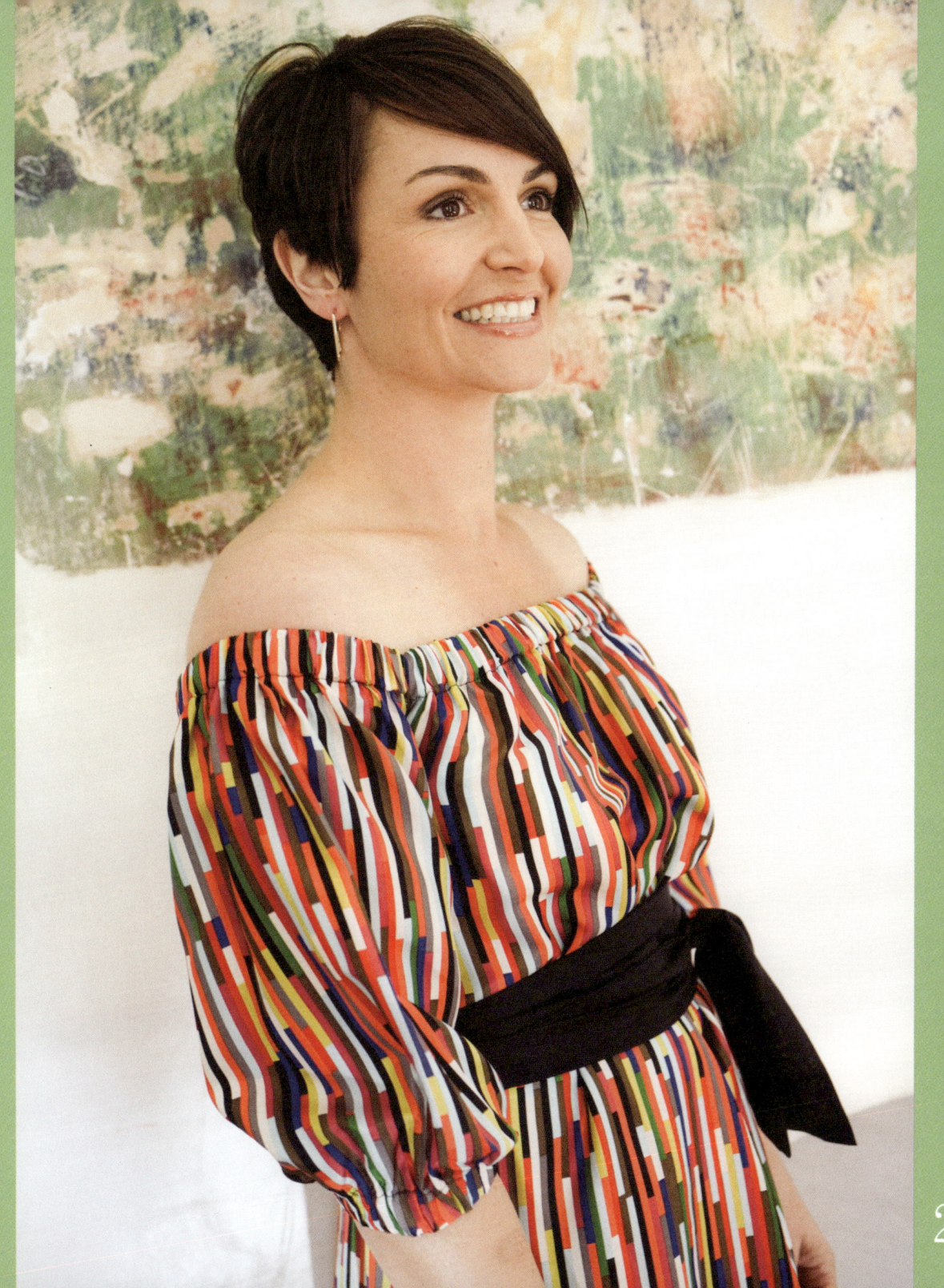

227

Acknowledgements

Thank you, team!

Although my name graces the cover, this book really is a team effort.
I am especially pleased to have completed it with my publisher and good
friend, Jill Brown. Jill had a vision for the book from the start and has
overseen the project with her creative eye. Jill, I can't thank you enough
and couldn't be happier with the end result.

A thousand thanks to the team Jill assembled. Jill, Helen Cooney,
Heather Curdie and Catherine Hill did a fabulous job editing my
words and being creative with titles and layout; Mary Louise Brammer
created the simply gorgeous design; Kiren Chang took the beautiful
photographs; Annebelle van Tongeren dressed me in glamorous style for
the shoot; and Belinda Weber did a lovely job with my hair and makeup.
I am also grateful for the dedication and enthusiasm given to my book
from the production, sales and marketing folks at Random House
Australia, and a special big thank you goes to my delightful publicist,
Claire Rose.

I am indebted to Sammie Coryton for agreeing to write recipes for me
despite moving back to London and having a full-time project of her
own. Sammie, I love your food, you were inspiring to work with and
I hope we can do so again. Thank you also to my wonderful literary
agent, Philippa Sandall, who dots the i's, crosses the t's and thinks of all
the things that I don't when it comes to the paperwork.

Thank you to all the women who took the time to complete my survey
and share their stories. Your insights were all-important and have
enriched this book enormously.

Finally, to my husband, Michael, and the many friends and family who
have endured months (for some, years) of me sounding out ideas and
brain-storming title suggestions – thank you all for putting up with me!

228

Notes

Chakravarthy, M. V. & Booth, F. W. (2004), *Eating, exercise, and 'thrifty' genotypes: connecting the dots toward an evolutionary understanding of modern chronic diseases. Journal of Applied Physiology,* 96: 3–10

Egger, G. J., Vogels, N. & Westerterp, K. R. (2001), *Estimating historical changes in physical activity levels. Medical Journal of Australia,* 175: 635–6

Gilbert, Elizabeth (2006), *Eat Pray Love.* Viking

Haskvitz, Sylvia (2005), *Eat by Choice, Not by Habit.* PuddleDancer Press

Kausman, Rick (1998), *If Not Dieting Then What?.* Allen & Unwin

O'Keefe, J. H. & Cordain, L. (2004), *Cardiovascular Disease Resulting from a Diet and Lifestyle at Odds With Our Paleolithic Genome: How to Become a 21st-Century Hunter-Gatherer. Mayo Clinic Proceedings,* 79:101–8

Pollan, Michael (2008), *In Defence of Food: the Myth of Nutrition and the Pleasures of Eating.* Allen Lane

Rappaport, Leon (2003), *How We Eat: Appetite, Culture and the Psychology of Food.* ECW Press

Rozin, P., Fischler, C., Imada, S., Sarubin, A. & Wrzesniewski, A. (1999), *Attitudes to food and the role of food in life in the USA, Japan, Flemish Belgium and France: possible implications for the diet-health debate. Appetite,* 33: 163–80

Saris, W. H., Blair, S. N., van Baak, M. A., et al. (2003). *How much physical activity is enough to prevent unhealthy weight gain? Outcome of the IASO 1st Stock Conference and consensus statement. Obesity Reviews,* 4: 101–14

Urbszat, D., Herman, C. P. & Polivy, J. (2002). *Eat, drink and be merry, for tomorrow we diet: effects of anticipated deprivation on food intake in restrained and unrestrained eaters. Journal of Abnormal Psychology,* 111(2): 396–401

Wansink, B., Payne, C. R. & Chandon, P. (2007). *Internal and external cues of meal cessation: the French paradox redux? Obesity Reviews,* 15 (12): 2920–4

An Ebury Press book
Published by Random House Australia Pty Ltd
Level 3, 100 Pacific Highway, North Sydney NSW 2060
www.randomhouse.com.au

First published by Ebury Press in 2009

Addresses for companies within the Random House Group can be found at
www.randomhouse.com.au/offices

National Library of Australia
Cataloguing-in-Publication Entry

McMillan Price, Joanna.
Inner health outer beauty.

ISBN 978 1 74166 806 3 (pbk.)

Diet.
Food habits.
Health.

613.7

Cover and internal design by Marylouise Brammer
Photography © Kiren Photography
Internal illustrations and patterns are from *Floral Design* (Dover Publications),
        except those in chapters 2 and 5, which are from *Indian Textile Prints* (The Pepin Press/
        Agile Rabbit editions)
Printed and bound by 1010 Printing International Limited

10 9 8 7 6 5 4 3 2 1

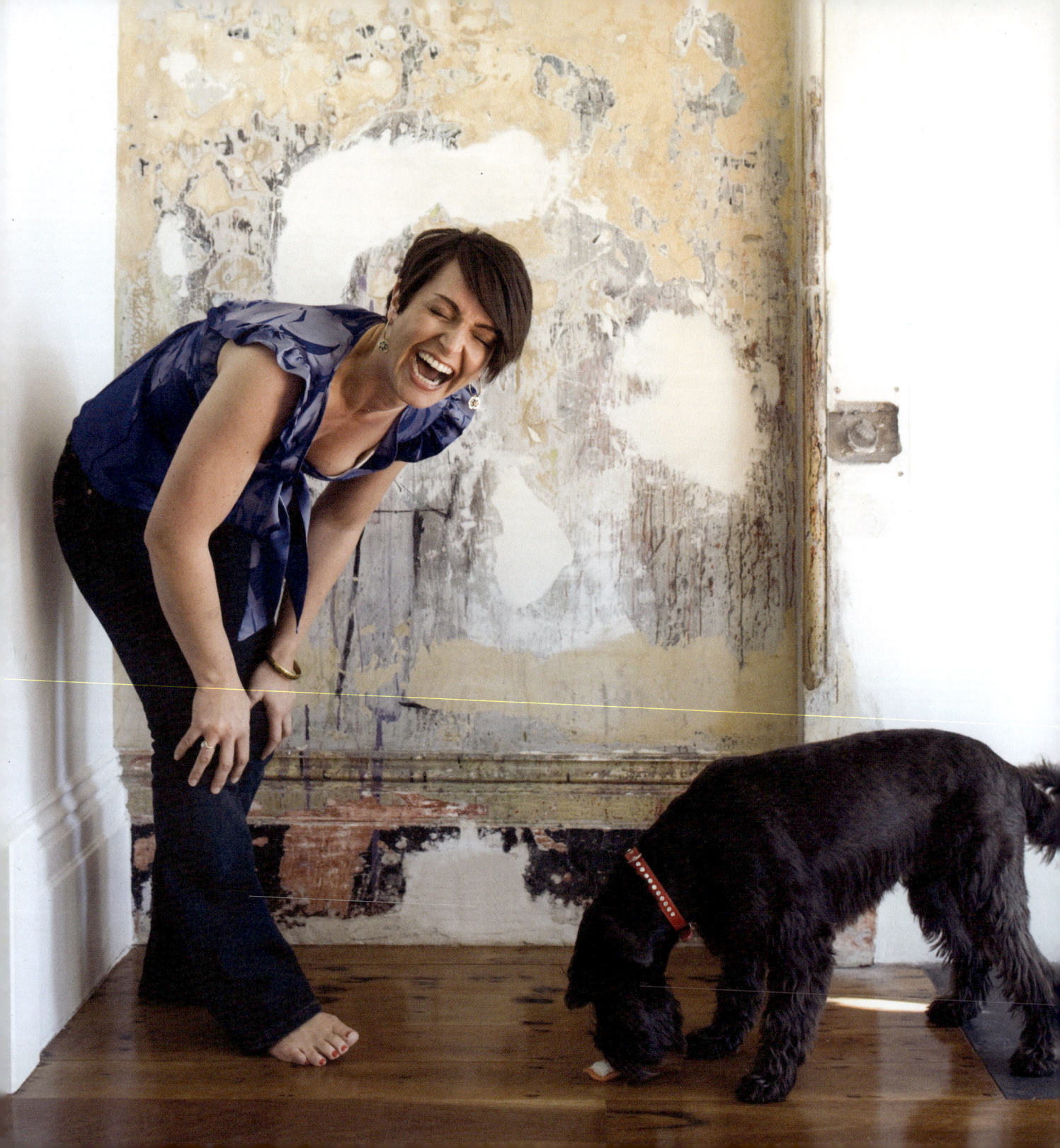